GOOD

...boost vitality...

MOOD

...beat the blues...

FOOD

...stay healthy...

GOOD

...boost vitality...

MOOD

...beat the blues...

FOOD

...stay healthy...

michael van straten

CASSELL&CO

Dedication

This book is dedicated to a remarkable woman who would have now been my adopted mother-in-law if she were still alive. Ruth Pearce was the epitome of someone who triumphed in the face of disaster, who overcame seemingly insurmountable health problems and who was an object lesson to everyone who knew her. Just being in Ruth's company was a guarantee of good mood, good conversation and good humour. She was always a tonic.

First published in the United Kingdom
in 2001 by Cassell & Co

A CIP catalogue record for this book is available from the British Library.

ISBN 0304 356204

Design: The Senate
Managing editor: Hilary Lumsden
Editor: Jamie Ambrose

Printed and bound by L.E.G.O in Italy

Cassell & Co
Wellington House
125 Strand
London WC2R 0BB

Contents

INTRODUCTION

There is a powerful connection between mood and food, yet surprisingly few people realize that this link exists. The mood-food connection is an everyday experience for most people, one that can be positive or negative. How is it possible, then, not to be aware of the intricate relationship between these two factors which have such a powerful influence on our lives?

After all, who hasn't enjoyed the elevated mood that follows a good meal in good company, or the awful depression that goes with a hangover after too much alcohol? Who hasn't felt the almost instant sharpening of concentration and alertness that follows a cup of strong black coffee, or fought the irritability, bad temper and forgetfulness that occur from going too long without food? I suspect few readers of this book have not been through these ups and downs, yet very few of them will have made the direct connection.

This is all the more surprising, considering the fact that, when they're feeling low, most people reach instinctively for the 'quick-fix' of high-sugar foods such as chocolate, biscuits or cakes, but these really are the nutritional recipe for disaster. Yes, they do provide a sudden leap of sugar to the bloodstream, which in turn offers a fairly instant boost of physical and mental energy. However, in order to cope with this rapid rise in blood sugar, your body releases a surge of insulin. Once the extra sugar has been converted into energy, the surplus insulin turns its attention to the residual sugar in the bloodstream and starts to break that down, too. The end result is a see-saw existence in which you satisfy your sugar and energy craving only to find that, by the end of half an hour or so, your blood sugar drops back to the level at which the sugar cravings return.

When patients in my surgery complain of repeated mood swings, I'm fairly certain that examining their dietary habits will reveal the cause.

This could include anything from poor nutrition or irregular eating to a huge dependence on high-sugar snacks and sweetened tea, coffee or cola drinks just to get them through the day. The solution to their problems, of course, is better eating habits and more use of good mood foods such as those described in this book.

The recipes in the following chapters are compiled from ingredients that have a known and proven impact on emotional conditions. The strength of that impact, however, also depends on mixing appropriate types of food – meat, fish, vegetables, salads, starchy foods, sweet fruits, nuts and seeds – with specific herbs and spices that have a positive action on mental and emotional states.

Take basil, for instance. It's one of nature's great mood-boosters, fostering calm and peaceful feelings. Likewise, sage has been used since ancient times to improve concentration and brain function, and it's no coincidence that rosemary is used as the herb of remembrance, as it specifically improves short-term memory function. Mint lifts the spirits, while chamomile calms them down. Nutmeg makes you feel happy, while ginger is a mental stimulant. Scented geranium promotes sleep; marjoram provides a wake-up call; myrtle and saffron are both aphrodisiacs; and lavender is a romantic mood-enhancer.

Whatever your mood or whatever you'd like it to be, you will find an appropriate recipe for it in this book. Use these dishes to create special moods for special occasions, or simply to provide you with a food idea that will change negative attitudes into positive ones. After all, a wealth of evidence shows beyond doubt that people with positive outlooks have stronger immune systems and lead healthier lives. *Good Mood Food* is designed for those who strive for such positivism.

HOW TO USE THIS BOOK

You can use this book to help create the mood you want, to get out of the mood you're in or to maintain your emotional status quo – whichever is appropriate. *Good Mood Food* provides the most pleasant, easily accessible and cheapest therapy you'll ever find. This book will help keep you sane, emotionally stable and out of the (often expensive) hands of therapists.

Quite simply, food *is* therapy. With the help of the information in this book, you can influence, change and manipulate your physical and emotional well-being simply by choosing the appropriate recipe. This is not a new or even controversial idea. More than 2,000 years ago, Hippocrates said that man should let his food be his medicine, and his medicine be his food; this statement is as true today as it was then. *Good Mood Food* provides the opportunity to put ancient theory into modern practice and discover for yourself just how well it works.

It is important, however, that you approach these therapeutic food remedies with some common sense. For example, if you've suffered from chronic fatigue for 12 months, you're not likely to be bounding with energy after one bowl of Sorrel-Leiki Soup (page 17), a dish of Smoky Pasta (page 20) or a succulent portion of Fantastic Figs (page 25) – all recipes from the 'Vitality Foods' chapter. If you have a chronic problem, then to get the best out of this book you will need to base your regular diet on the whole range of foods that are appropriate to you. Yes, you'll notice some changes very quickly, but in order to overcome any long-standing nutritional deficiencies that may have contributed to your health problem, it may take two or three months before you see any results.

The situation is different when you're facing more immediate problems such as a vital interview, a major exam or a key business meeting. In situations like these, you need instant results, and you'll find recipes that provide them in the 'Brain Foods' chapter. There's Minty Potato Soup (page 33), for example, with its calming and stress-busting volatile oils, or Spaghettini à la Vongole (page 35), which makes a perfect fishy brain food to sharpen your concentration. You can even indulge yourself with a helping of Granny Bly's Ice Cream (page 40), which combines the perfect brain food — honey — and the calming aroma of lavender.

For the occasional troubled sleeper, using recipes from the 'Snooze Foods' section will provide instant relief. If you're a chronic insomniac, you will need to use these recipes on a regular basis as an aid to solving long-term sleep problems. Start with an evening glass of Super Snoozer (page 48), or try a bowl of Lullaby Lettuce Soup (page 49). As a light supper, how about a portion of Sleepy Sesame Chicken (page 53), full of calming B vitamins? For a real treat that will usher you off to the land of nod, try the DDG Chocolate Crêpes (page 56). The luscious mixture of cocoa and chocolate liqueur gives you the benefit of soothing theobromine and a modest amount of alcohol — just try and stay awake long enough to finish it.

Whether it's stress or sensitivity you want to relieve, or whether you want to foster feelings of sensuality. . . whatever your mood problem, you should find something to help you in *Good Mood Food*. It even includes a selection of special diets for special needs, which range from a selection of 'Stress-Buster Diets' (page 152) to the 'Happy Weight-Loss Diet' (page 154) and the 'Ultimate Aphrodisiac Diet' (page 156). Finally, the 'Good Mood A–Z' (page 138) will guide you through a range of problems, listing the most appropriate foods and recipes to choose in order to sort them out. Whatever the reason you use this book, use it to enjoy the therapeutic benefits of cooking and the enormous pleasure of eating good mood food, preferably with those closest to you. Most recipes serve four, but those in the 'Sexy Foods' section are, naturally, made for two.

GOOD

FO

MOOD
OD

VITALITY FOODS

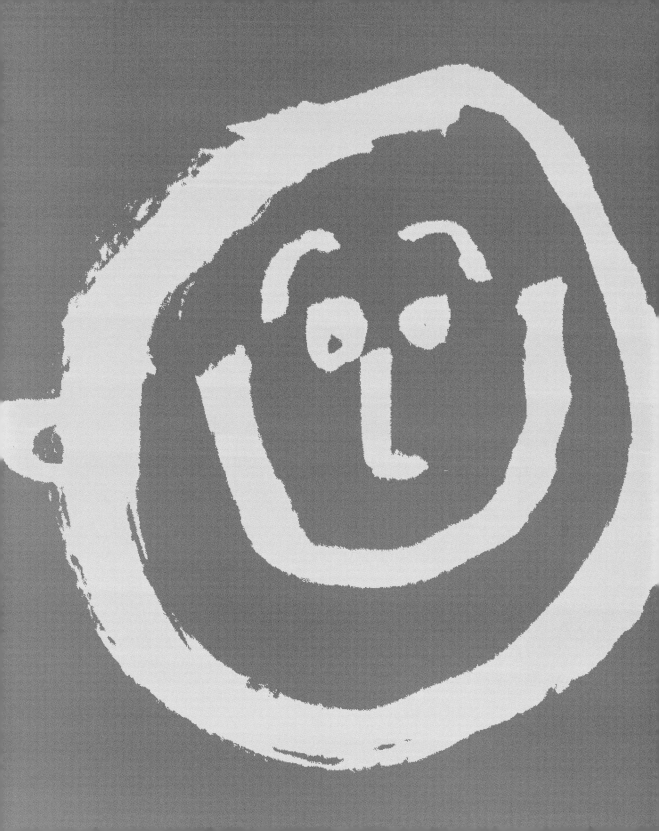

VITALITY FOODS

Vitality means physical or mental vigour and the ability to live, grow and thrive. If you're operating at less-than-peak levels, then stop here. This chapter provides recipes that include the most vital of foods – vital not only for their rich content of essential nutrients, but also for their renowned and revered abilities to stimulate, restore and invigorate flagging energy.

Of course, if you're feeling a bit low, you don't want to waste energy on difficult or complicated recipes. Don't worry: all of the recipes in this section are easy to follow. The chapter begins with a super-vitality juice that requires nothing more than putting the ingredients through a juicer. For this minimal amount of effort, you get an instant energy boost to drink any time of the day or night.

You will also receive an incredible immune boost from easy recipes such as Sorrel-Leiki Soup (page 17), which offers energy from potatoes and the protective benefits of leeks and onions. Perfect for a convalescent recovering from illness, but just as wonderful for the business high-flyer who needs to raise vitality after a gruelling week.

In addition to including recipes such as these in your diet, you need to avoid excessive consumption of over-refined, starchy foods that deplete your body's vital energy. Top of the hit-list should be refined sugar, which no one needs and the amounts of which you can halve in virtually every published recipe – except in this book, where they have already been reduced. This is because sugar contains no nutrients, just empty calories, which is why foods high in sugar give you an instant but short-lived energy boost followed by a sinking, low-vitality drop in blood-sugar levels.

All the recipes in this section are rich in the vitality-enhancing natural ingredients that the body needs in order to maintain peak vitality as well as to generate extra reserves at time of need. One of the main requirements is an abundance of slow-release energy that comes from complex carbohydrates such as pasta, wholemeal bread, rice, polenta and potatoes. For this reason, another key to increasing and maintaining good levels of vitality is to ignore the myth that bread, rice, potatoes and pasta are fattening; they're not. They are great vitality foods, and are only fattening if you do the wrong things with them.

From now on, then, just decrease the butter on your bread – not the bread itself. Eat potatoes boiled, baked in their skins or roasted in the oven with a little olive oil and rosemary. Eat pasta in the traditional Italian way: with extra-virgin olive oil and plenty of garlic – a super-vitality booster in its own right. Use tomato sauce with tuna or smoked mackerel, eat rice any way you like, but don't smother dishes in cheese, cream or butter.

Nuts and seeds play an essential part in any vitality plan, as they supply slow-release energy together with protein for stamina. They also provide essential minerals – especially zinc, one of nature's great fatigue-fighters – and a rich supply of vitamin E, which protects the heart and circulatory system.

Energy can also be indulgent, thank heavens, which is why this chapter ends with two fantastic desserts that will tickle the taste buds of the most dedicated sweet-lover. Tart's Delight (page 24), for example, is made with sweet, succulent cherries which ooze vitality, thanks to their high potassium and vitamin C content. Meanwhile, Fantastic Figs (page 25) features the most succulent and sensuous of fruits. You'll get a great lift from the brandy, lots of protein and calcium from the goats' cheese and an enormous boost to your vitality and natural immunity just from the pleasure offered by this oh-so-simple recipe. Enjoy!

PEAR-POWER PUNCH

Vitality means a strong heart and boundless energy. That's what you get from this wonderful juice: instant energy from the natural sugars in the pears, which also supply special fibre to lower cholesterol and protect the heart. There is also plenty of slow-release energy and protein from the almonds, which generate a subtle, bitter-sweet flavour that revitalizes the palate.

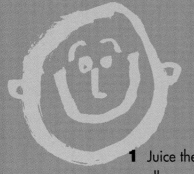

2 firm **Conference pears**
2 **celery sticks**, with leaves
115g ᵒʳ 4oz fresh **young spinach leaves**
1 tbsp ground **almonds**
mint leaves, for garnish

1 Juice the pears, celery sticks and young spinach in an all-purpose juicer.
2 Stir in the ground almonds.
3 Adjust the consistency, if necessary, by adding mineral water.
4 Pour into glasses, decorate with mint leaves, and serve.

SORREL-LEIKI SOUP

Aunt Leiki was the famous soup-maker in my mother's family. This was her recipe for anyone needing a vitality boost, whether hungover, convalescing or just feeling below par. The onions and leeks provide a surge to the immune system, the sorrel supplies vital iron and the vegetable stock offers masses of minerals.

450g or 1lb **potatoes**, peeled and diced
1.2 litres or 40fl oz **organic vegetable stock**
2 medium **onions**, chopped
3 medium **leeks**, finely sliced
4 tbsps **rape-seed oil**
2 large bunches of **sorrel** (or rocket), cleaned and finely chopped
300ml or 10fl oz **crème fraîche** or **single cream**

1 In a large saucepan, simmer the potatoes in the stock until tender.
2 In a separate saucepan, sweat the onions and leeks gently in the oil.
3 Pour the onion mixture into the potatoes and stock. Add the sorrel, reserving two tablespoons for garnish. Remove from heat and allow to infuse for 15 minutes.
4 Using a food processor or mouli, liquidize the mixture.
5 Add the crème fraîche or cream and stir well.
6 Reheat (but do not boil) to serve hot, or chill and serve cold.
7 Garnish with the finely chopped sorrel leaves.

CHEF'S NOTE: Rape-seed oil is used here instead of extra-virgin olive oil, which would overpower the exquisite taste of this delicate soup.

SAVOURY POLENTA CAKE

Here's another simple, wonderful and revitalizing dish. Although its energy comes from the starchy polenta and the protein found in the cheese, its real benefits are derived from the herbs. Rocket has been used as a tonic medicine since Elizabethan times, chervil serves as a blood purifier, chives reduce cholesterol and parsley provides cleansing properties.

1 litre ^{or} 34fl oz **organic vegetable stock**
200g ^{or} 7oz **coarse polenta**
1 large handful of **rocket**, roughly torn
85g ^{or} 3oz **Parmesan cheese**
2 tsps **parsley**, chopped
2 tsps **chervil**, chopped
2 tsps **chives**, chopped
salt and freshly ground **black pepper**, to taste

1 In a large saucepan, bring the vegetable stock to a boil.
2 Add the polenta gradually, stirring to prevent any lumps from forming.
3 Simmer for about 30 minutes, stirring frequently, until the mixture comes away from the pan.
4 Stir in the rocket, cheese and herbs. Season to taste.
5 Pour the mixture into a greased, square baking dish and bake at 180°C ^{or} 350°F ^{or} gas mark 4 for 20 minutes, until firm and golden.

SQUASH, TOMATOES & STEW

Boost your vitality with the masses of carbohydrate and high-protein content of red Camargue rice. It looks terrific with the pale gold of squash or pumpkin, the rich orange sweet potato and the green spinach. This stew overflows with vitalizing vitamins, minerals and heart-protecting lycopene.

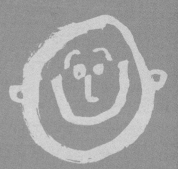

115g or 4oz **Camargue rice**
1 medium **onion**, chopped
4 tbsps **extra-virgin olive oil**
1 tsp **cumin**
½ tsp **cinnamon**
1 small **squash**, such as **butternut**, or a chunk of **pumpkin**, deseeded, peeled and diced
1 small **sweet potato**, peeled, diced and parboiled
225g or 8oz can **chopped tomatoes**
300ml or 10fl oz **organic vegetable stock**
1 tsp **garam masala**
200g or 7oz **baby leaf spinach**

1 Cook the rice as per instructions (Camargue takes about 30 minutes).
2 Sweat the onion in the oil. Add the cumin and cinnamon and cook for two minutes.
3 Soften the squash and potato with the onion for four to five minutes.
4 Add the stock and tomatoes. Simmer until nearly tender.
5 Stir in the garam masala and add the spinach on top. Cover and simmer for three minutes, until the spinach wilts into a green covering.
6 Serve the vegetables on a bed of rice.

SMOKY PASTA

Pasta and oily fish: you couldn't imagine more vital foods. Energy, protein, vitamin C, bioflavonoids, the fantastic flavours of tart grapefruit and the smooth oiliness of smoked salmon and mackerel make this salad an all-time winner as a starter, light lunch or late supper.

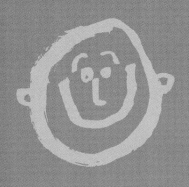

175g or 6oz **penne, organic** if possible
1 medium **courgette**, finely sliced
115g or 4oz **French beans**, finely snipped
100ml or 3½ fl oz freshly squeezed **grapefruit juice**
3 tbsps **extra-virgin olive oil**
1 **grapefruit**, segmented
280g or 10oz **smoked mackerel**
55g or 2oz **smoked salmon**
2 tbsps **flat-leaf parsley**, finely chopped
2 tbsps **chives**, finely snipped

1 Cook the pasta according to the instructions on the package.
2 In a pan, simmer the courgette and beans until just tender.
3 Mix the oil and grapefruit juice. Stir into the pasta and cool.
4 Flake the mackerel. Chop the smoked salmon.
5 Combine all the ingredients. Season to taste, and sprinkle with the herbs.

TANTALIZING TUNA

Boundless vitality is yours with this combination of lentils, protein-rich tuna and almonds, and the carrot's super-boosting and protective carotenoids. Add the calcium from milk, B vitamins from the egg and all the heart-protective properties of oily fish and onions for a dish that will keep your pulse ticking like a Swiss watch.

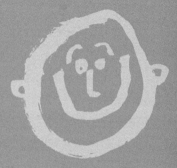

115g or 4oz **lentils**
3 large **spring onions**, finely chopped
(including the green leaves)
3 tbsps **extra-virgin olive oil**
1 **egg**
150ml or 5fl oz **milk**
175g or 6oz can **tuna**, in brine, drained before use
1 medium **carrot**, grated
55g or 2oz flaked **almonds**

1 In a covered saucepan, boil the lentils in water, stirring occasionally, until tender – approximately 20 to 30 minutes; check to make sure they don't dry out.
2 Soften the spring onions in the oil.
3 Beat the egg into the milk.
4 Combine the lentils, tuna, carrot, spring onions and egg mixture. Place in a shallow oven-proof casserole dish. Sprinkle over the almonds and cook at 200°C or 400°F or gas mark 6 for 30 minutes.

FISHY RICE & PEAS

Unlike traditional West Indian rice and peas made with black-eyed peas, this dish uses green peas, an equally good source of energy and protein. As well as offering minerals and protein in the fish, carbohydrate in the rice and vitality-boosting spices in the curry, it's full of flavour, providing a plateful of delicious vitality food.

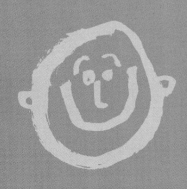

1 small **onion**, sliced
1 **garlic** clove, chopped
3 tbsps **extra-virgin olive oil**
2 tsps **curry powder**
400ml or 14fl oz **organic vegetable stock**
150ml or 5fl oz **coconut milk**
115g or 4oz **rice**
115g or 4oz fillet each of **cod** and **haddock**, cut into chunks
200g or 7oz **frozen peas**

1 In a saucepan, sweat the onion and garlic in the oil.
2 Sprinkle in the curry powder, add two tablespoons of the stock and mix thoroughly.
3 Mix the coconut milk with the remaining stock. Add the stock and rice to the onion mixture and simmer until the liquid is almost absorbed – approximately 15 to 20 minutes.
4 Mix in the fish and peas, and cook until all ingredients are tender – approximately five minutes.

NUTTY CHICKEN

I first ate chicken cooked with pine nuts in 1964, in southern Portugal, where it is a traditional peasant dish. The combined aroma of garlic, allspice and peppercorns will get your taste buds zinging before the first bite, and every ingredient in this dish will boost your vitality.

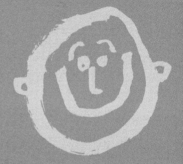

4 on-the-bone, skinless **organic chicken thighs**
3 tbsps **peanut oil**
1 large **sweet onion**, finely chopped
2 **garlic** cloves, finely chopped
1 slice of **organic stone-ground bread**,
   removed and cubed
8 **peppercorns**, crushed
1 tsp **allspice**
55g or 2oz **pine nuts**
200ml or 7fl oz **dry red wine**

1 In a large skillet, brown the chicken in the oil; remove and keep warm.
2 Turn down the heat, add the onion and garlic and cook until softened.
3 Add the bread cubes and fry at a higher heat until golden brown.
4 Mix the crushed peppercorns with the allspice, then add the spices and pine nuts to the bread cubes and fry for one minute, stirring constantly. Add the wine.
5 Place the chicken thighs in an oven-proof casserole dish. Add the wine mixture and cook at 200°C or 400°F or gas mark 6 for 40 minutes, adding more wine or water if necessary.

TART'S DELIGHT

Cherries are not only one of the most delicious of all fruits, they're also one of the few remaining seasonal delights. Super-rich in vitamin C, potassium and cancer-fighting phytochemicals, they are one of nature's great vitality foods. Extra energy comes from the ground almonds, along with protein and iron from the eggs. Enjoy this one with a clear conscience!

1 pack of **shortcrust pastry**, or ready-made **pastry crust**
450g or 1lb **fresh red cherries** or **canned fruit**, drained and rinsed
115g or 4oz **caster sugar**
2 **eggs**
115g or 4oz ground **almonds**

1 If using uncooked pastry, bake it blind in a 21cm or 9-inch flan tin for 10 minutes at 190°C or 375°F or gas mark 5.
2 Stone the cherries, if necessary, then simmer them gently for five minutes in just enough water to cover.
3 Sieve the sugar to prevent lumps. Whisk the eggs and mix in the ground almonds and sugar until the mixture has a paste-like consistency.
4 Arrange the cherries in the pastry case. Pour over the almond paste. Bake at 200°C or 400°F or gas mark 5–6 for 30 minutes.

CHEF'S NOTE: This recipe will easily serve four, and is equally delicious cold the next day.

FANTASTIC FIGS

Fresh figs are the ultimate succulent, sensuous, delicious, vitality-boosting fruit. They're rich in betacarotene, iron, potassium and cancer-fighting phytochemicals, which, together with their natural sugar content, provide an instant boost. Add the health benefits of calcium in the goats' cheese and the circulation boost from the brandy, and you have a dessert that provides pure pleasure with no pain.

6 ripe **figs**
4 tbsps **brandy**
225g or 8oz **soft goats' cheese**, a cylindrical
variety cut into 12 equal slices

1 Slice the figs lengthways. Arrange them in a heat-proof dish so that they fit snugly.
2 Spoon the brandy equally over each fruit.
3 Top each fig half with a slice of goats' cheese.
4 Place under a pre-heated hot grill for five minutes.

VITALITY HERB

GARLIC

Originally a native of China and Asia, garlic has been used in traditional medicine as a powerful antiseptic, antifungal and antibacterial. From the *hajo blanco* (white garlic soup) of southern Spain to the onion and garlic soup of East Anglia, this herb is famed for its therapeutic value in the treatment of chest infections. In fact, the combination of garlic and onion, both members of the allium family, is probably the starting point for more traditional soup, stew and casserole recipes than any other in the world.

However, it is the most modern scientific research that has secured garlic's place as a vitality booster. Evidence has shown that it lowers cholesterol, reduces blood pressure and decreases the stickiness of blood, thus minimizing the risk of heart disease and strokes. It therefore increases the likelihood of a longer, healthier and physically more active and vital life.

To get the maximum vitality boost and the benefits of the protective strength of garlic, eat the equivalent of one whole clove a day. Don't worry about the smell — that's what does the most good. The odour is caused by the sulphur compounds allicin and alliin, both of which may help prevent cancers of the digestive tract. When using garlic in cooking, allow it to stand for five to ten minutes after chopping: exposure to the air causes oxidation, which releases the healing chemicals.

Sadly, some people don't like the taste of this wonderful plant, and there are those whose digestions won't tolerate it. For these unfortunates, there is the option of taking garlic in tablet form. Many varieties exist, including oil capsules, deodorized versions and expensive, oriental, 'aged' garlic pills. I recommend avoidance of all but those tablets that are made from the whole dried bulb and contain a standardized dose in every pill.

VITALITY SPICE

CINNAMON

Cinnamon is one of the earliest of spices to be traded anywhere in the world, and is one of the oldest aromatic plants on record. While it was mentioned in the Old Testament, it was not 'officially' discovered by the West until sometime during the late 15th to early 16th centuries, in Sri Lanka.

This wonderfully aromatic spice is a member of the laurel family, and is made from the plant's dried bark. It can be used as a powder, in small pieces or in the form of wonderfully fragrant cinnamon sticks. The sticks are made by rolling layers of bark by hand to form the cylindrical shape, then repeatedly rolling them until the bark has completely dried out and turned the beautiful shade of reddish-brown that shares its name.

Besides adding its wonderful flavour to food, cinnamon is a vitality-boosting stimulant and tonic as well as an antiseptic. It is a great remedy for the exhaustion and general tiredness that often follow common infectious illnesses such as colds and flu. Immersing a stick into a hot toddy of boiling water, honey, lemon and whisky releases the volatile oil cinnamaldehyde, which not only has a tonic effect, but is also a gentle painkiller. Boiling a cinnamon stick in water makes a good inhalation for blocked sinuses and chesty coughs. Like ylang-ylang or patchouli, it is also considered to have aphrodisiac properties when used in aromatherapy.

In Britain, cinnamon is used mainly in sweet dishes, but in other parts of the world, it is just as popular in savoury foods, such as in traditional Middle Eastern rice dishes and the famous lamb tagine from Morocco.

BRAIN FOODS

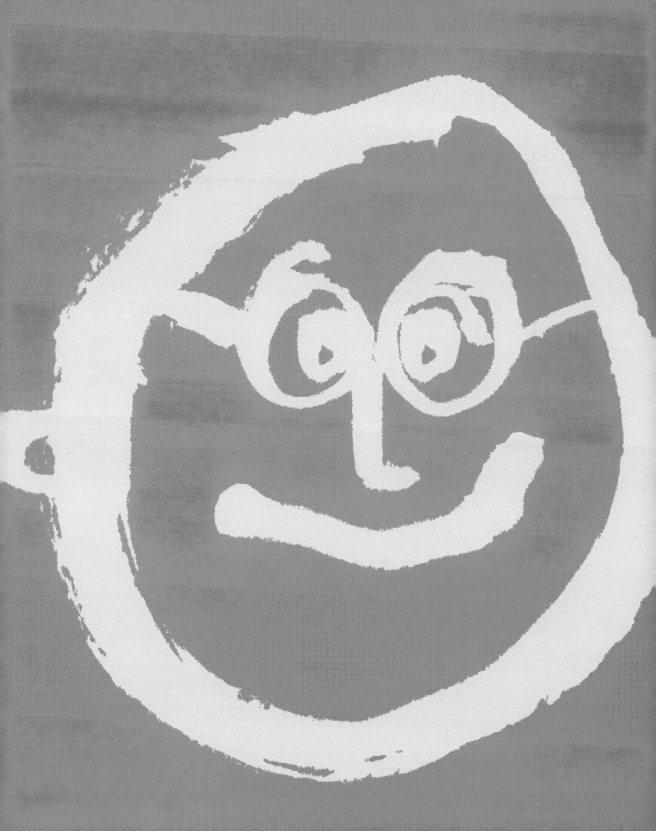

BRAIN FOODS

When granny said, 'Eat your fish: it will make you brainy', she wasn't far off the mark. All oily fish contain essential fatty acids, which makes them vital foods for any woman who is planning to have a baby, or who is pregnant or breastfeeding. Fatty acids form a major part of a developing baby's brain tissue, and there is now substantial evidence that women whose diets are low in fish oils have children who tend to have slower mental development. Yet it's not just oily fish that make good brain food; the protein in all types of fish provides some slow-release energy, which helps to keep a constant supply of blood sugar flowing to the brain. This is exactly what it needs in order to function consistently.

While all forms of protein make good nourishment for the brain, it is important to avoid animal proteins which contain large amounts of saturated fat. Poultry, game and lean, free-range beef are ideal, especially if you remove all visible fat and avoid eating the skin on chicken, duck or turkey. Saturated fat can lead to raised cholesterol levels, fatty deposits in the arteries and narrowing of the blood vessels which supply the brain – often the first step towards declining brain function.

For the same reasons, wholegrain cereals, all the beans, garlic, leeks and onions should be regular ingredients in any cerebral eating plan. All of these foods help rid the body of excessive amounts of cholesterol. This in turn helps keep the levels of this damaging deposit healthily low, ensuring the maintenance of an adequate and continuous blood supply which carries essential nutrients to every cell in the brain.

Modest amounts of alcohol are good news for your brain, too. The high levels of antioxidants that prevent brain cell damage are a major component of red wine, so a couple of glasses a day are a great ally in the maintenance of good mental function.

Alcohol itself is also valuable, whether it comes from wine, beer, spirits or liqueurs. In small amounts, it has the effect of opening up the tiniest blood vessels at the end of the circulatory system and improving blood flow to the brain – if you consume just two or three glasses of wine, or two or three pub measures of spirits, or up to two pints of beer a day. The bad news is that once you exceed these quantities, alcohol has exactly the opposite effect and makes minute vessels contract, depriving the brain of blood and leading to rapid deterioration in mental ability.

Herbs and spices also have a vital role as brain foods, and they work in various ways. Some herbs, such as basil, nutmeg, lemon balm and coriander, affect mood and emotion; others have a more direct impact on mental function. The two most powerful of these are sage, synonymous with wisdom, and rosemary, linked with improved memory since ancient times. The most important spice is chilli, which opens up the tiniest blood vessels, leading to an almost instant rush of blood to the head. (This accounts for the beads of sweat on the forehead within seconds of your first mouthful of a strong chilli con carne.) Ginger comes a close second, and will also provide quick brain stimulation whether taken as tea, a sprinkle of powder or fresh in a stir-fry.

Because of today's longer life expectancy, the maintenance of good brain function is more crucial than ever. By accentuating the positive aspects of diet and eliminating the negatives, you dramatically increase your chances of maintaining mental agility well into old age. Yet food alone isn't enough. The brain is like any part of the body: if you don't use it, you lose it. Keep it active by reading, conversation, crossword puzzles, learning a few lines of poetry and memory games. Most important is the process of calculation. Doing sums is the ultimate key to mental prowess – just following these recipes and working out the quantities is a start. For your brain's sake, get cooking.

CHOC-A-LOT SMOOTHIE

Here's a brain booster that mixes chocolate, containing
the brain stimulant theobromine, with myristicin,
a mood-enhancing chemical found in nutmeg.
Combined with folic acid, magnesium, potassium
and fruit sugars in banana, this smoothie makes
a delicious way of boosting anyone's brain power.

300ml or 10fl oz plain **bio-yoghurt**
1 heaped tbsp **organic chocolate powder**
1 **banana**, chopped
a sprinkle of **nutmeg**, mixed with an extra pinch
of **chocolate powder**

1 Place the first three ingredients in a food processor or blender and
blend until smooth.

2 Pour into glasses, and sprinkle with nutmeg and chocolate powder
for a final touch.

CHEF'S NOTE: Bio- (or live) yoghurts are always preferable to use in any
recipe, as they contain huge amounts of living pro-biotic, or beneficial,
bacteria. These 'bugs' are protective, aid digestion and also boost the
body's natural immunity. If you're watching your weight, use low-fat
bio-yoghurt instead.

MINTY POTATO SOUP

In spite of a little garlic, the overwhelming flavour and aroma of this delicate broth is that of mint, a natural breath freshener. And it's the mint and its volatile oils – menthol and menthone – which make this soup a great mood-enhancer, too. The coumarins in celery add to its stress-busting benefits.

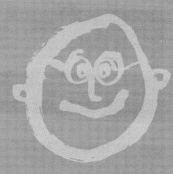

1 **onion**, finely chopped
½ a **garlic** clove, finely chopped
4 tbsps **extra-virgin olive oil**
1 whole bunch of **celery**, with leaves
1 large **potato**, diced
850ml ᵒʳ 29fl oz **organic vegetable stock**
1 small handful of **mint**, finely chopped

1 In a large saucepan, sweat the onion and garlic in the oil.
2 Chop the celery sticks and add to the saucepan, reserving the leaves. Cover and cook gently for 20 minutes.
3 Add the potatoes and stock, and simmer until tender.
4 Using a food processor or mouli, liquidize until smooth.
5 Serve sprinkled with chopped mint and whole celery leaves.

EASY CHEESE FRITTATA

The natural chemical capsaicin in chillies provides a great boost to the circulatory system, increasing blood flow to the brain as well as to other parts of the body. B vitamins in the eggs are excellent brain food, while the cheese contains tryptophan, which encourages the release of brain-calming hormones. This recipe makes a perfect light supper: easy to cook and ready in minutes.

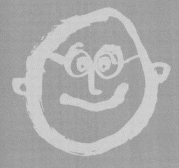

6 medium **eggs**
1 1/2 tbsps **flat-leaf parsley**, chopped
1 1/2 tbsps **chives**, chopped
2 tbsps **extra-virgin olive oil**
2 thin rashers of **back bacon**, finely snipped
225g or 8oz small **broccoli** florets, cut into quarters
1 fresh **red chilli**, deseeded and finely chopped
115g or 4oz **gruyère cheese**, grated

1 Beat together the eggs and herbs.
2 In a large skillet, heat the oil, add the bacon, broccoli and chilli and cook gently, stirring frequently, until the broccoli is tender – approximately 8 to ten minutes.
3 Mix the cheese into the egg mixture and pour over the broccoli and bacon mixture.
4 Cook over a medium heat for seven minutes, then finish cooking under a pre-heated grill for about three minutes.
5 Serve hot or cold.

SPAGHETTINI A LA VONGOLE

Oily fish is essential during pregnancy and breast-feeding for optimum brain development in babies. Even for adults, there is no doubt that all fish and shellfish are brain food. This classic Italian dish uses small clams, which have a high brain-boosting zinc and selenium content.

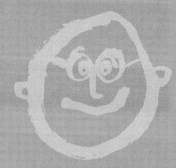

675g or 1½ lbs **clams**, rinsed thoroughly
225g or 8oz **spaghettini**
55g or 2oz unsalted **butter**
2 tbsps **extra-virgin olive oil**
1 small **onion**, finely chopped
2 **garlic** cloves, finely chopped
½ glass of **dry white wine**
1 large cup of **curly parsley**, finely chopped

1 Simmer the clams, covered, in half a cup of water until they open.
2 Remove the clams, strain their liquor through muslin and reserve.
3 Cook the pasta according to the instructions on the package.
4 In a large saucepan, sweat the onion and garlic in the butter and oil. Add the wine and clam liquor and boil for five minutes.
5 Add the clams, season to taste, then stir in the parsley. Pour over the pasta to serve.

CHEF'S NOTE: You can remove the clams from their shells, but I think this dish is much more appealing – and more fun to eat – if they're left in. This recipe is best made with dry pasta rather than fresh; choose your favourite.

WISE OLD FISH

It's no coincidence that the name of the herb and the word for a wise old person are the same: sage. Known and used since ancient times, its botanical name is *Salvia*, from the Latin meaning 'healing plant', and its brain-boosting properties are legendary. So what better than sage combined with fish for the ultimate brain-power dish?

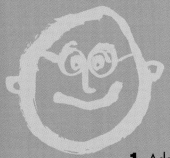

8 **sage leaves**, bruised and finely chopped
8 tbsps **extra-virgin olive oil**
2 middle fillets of **cod**, **haddock** or **hake**, skins on, each weighing about 175g or 6oz
2 **beef tomatoes**, finely sliced widthways
55g or 2oz **unsalted butter**

1 Add the sage leaves to two tablespoons of the oil and set aside.
2 Score the fish on the skin side, season all over and fry, skin-side down only, in the rest of the oil until crisp.
3 Transfer the fillets to an oven-proof dish and cook, skin-side down, at 230°C or 450°F or gas mark 8 until tender – approximately eight to ten minutes.
4 Fry the tomatoes gently in the butter for two minutes each side.
5 Serve the fish topped with tomatoes and drizzled with the sage oil.

HOT, HONEYED PRAWNS

Chilli again – this time green, but with the same capsaicin content, that stimulates blood flow to the brain. In addition, the lemon grass provides a mild sedative effect, coriander is a strong mood-enhancer and the prawns, like all shellfish, are an ultimate brain food.

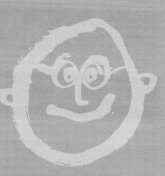

½ a **green chilli**
5cm or 2-inch piece of **lemon grass**, chopped
1 tbsp **coriander** leaf, roughly torn
2 tbsps **fish sauce**
2 tbsps **lime juice**
1 tbsp **runny honey**
100ml or 3½ fl oz **dry white wine**
280g or 10oz cooked **prawns**, with shells, well washed
3 tbsps **rape-seed oil**

1 Mix the first seven ingredients together.
2 Add the prawns, and mix carefully but thoroughly. Cover and place in a refrigerator to marinate for at least two hours.
3 Drain the prawns, reserving the marinade.
4 Heat the oil in a wok or deep frying pan until smoking and stir-fry the prawns for four to five minutes.
5 Remove from the wok, then add the marinade. Boil briskly for two minutes, then pour over the prawns. Serve with jasmine rice or other, flavoured rice.

POUSSIN PARCELS

With its high protein and vitamin B content, chicken really is food for the brain. This recipe combines chicken with the all-healing properties of cabbage and the strong, mood-enhancing effect of tarragon. It's unusual, simple and produces far more complex flavours than you'd imagine.

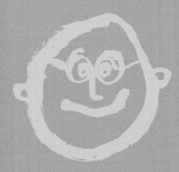

2 small **poussins**
4 sprigs of **tarragon**, finely chopped
2 rashers of **smoked bacon**
enough blanched **Savoy cabbage leaves** to wrap around each bird
3 **bay leaves**
5 whole **peppercorns**
a pinch of **sea salt**

1 Season the birds inside and out.
2 Place the tarragon inside each cavity and drape a rasher of bacon over each breast.
3 Wrap each bird with cabbage leaves and tie firmly with string.
4 Place the birds in a saucepan of cold water, along with the bay leaves, peppercorns and salt. Bring to a boil and simmer, covered, for 35 minutes.
5 Remove with a slotted spoon and serve on a bed of herb-flavoured rice.

SMART SHEPHERD'S PIE

You won't find many foolish shepherds. These wise men and women invented the shepherd's pie – originally made from cold, leftover lamb. Made with beef, this could be considered cottage pie, but with brain-enhancing protein and the extraordinary mental stimulus of sage, it's old-fashioned brain food for the real meat-lover – whatever the name.

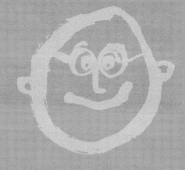

1 small **onion**, chopped
2 **garlic** cloves, chopped
150ml or 5fl oz **extra-virgin olive oil**
225g or 8oz lean **minced beef**
½ a **swede**, peeled and finely grated
300ml or 10fl oz hot **beef stock**
450g or 1lb **potatoes**, peeled and diced
a handful of **sage leaves**, finely chopped

1 Soften the onion and garlic in three tablespoons of the oil.
2 Add the beef and brown gently.
3 Stir in the grated swede and stock and transfer the mixture to an oven-proof casserole dish.
4 Boil the potatoes, drain, then dry thoroughly over a gentle heat. Mash them with the rest of the oil.
5 Stir in the sage leaves. Pile the potato mixture on top of the meat. Bake at 220°C or 425°F or gas mark 7 for 30 minutes.

CHEF'S NOTE: Dry the potatoes thoroughly before mashing to allow the flavours of the olive oil and sage to shine through.

GRANNY BLY'S ICE CREAM

Sadly, I never knew my own granny, but my oldest friend's grandmother was the epitome of a Victorian lady, with hat, gloves and the unmistakable fragrance of English lavender. I never smell this brain-enhancing herb without thinking of her. Honey has been used as brain food since the time of the ancient Egyptians, and makes a perfect partner for the lavender.

400ml ᵒʳ 14fl oz **Greek yoghurt**
125g ᵒʳ 4fl oz **honey**
1 tsp **vanilla extract**
300ml ᵒʳ 10fl oz **whipping cream**
lavender flowers, removed from 10 stalks

1 In a large bowl, mix all the ingredients together thoroughly.
2 Place in an ice cream maker and follow the instructions, or pour the mixture into a shallow, freezer-proof container and whisk every 30 to 45 minutes until creamy and just frozen – about two hours.

CHEF'S NOTE: It's hardly worth making ice cream for just two people. These quantities serve six to eight – and, of course, ice cream keeps well in the freezer. Remove one hour before serving.

BRAZILIAN BRANDY PUDDING

Sounds exotic, doesn't it? So put aside those memories of school dinners and take a chance on this fabulously posh tapioca. Made from the root of the manioc (cassava) shrub, which is native to Central and South America, tapioca is the staple energy food of the rainforest indians. This high-starch, ultra-low-fat dessert really will get those brain cells buzzing.

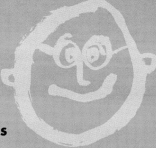

25g or 1oz **tapioca**
300ml or 10fl oz **milk**
1 tbsp **honey**
2 tbsps **apricot brandy**
25g or 1oz **dried apricots**, finely snipped
4 tbsps **organic fromage frais**
1 small punnet of **raspberries** or other **fresh berries**

1 In a large saucepan, warm the tapioca and milk gently and bring to a boil, stirring constantly.
2 Simmer until thick and creamy – around 10 to 15 minutes.
3 Stir in the honey, brandy and apricots.
4 Pour into an oven-proof dish and bake at 200°C or 400°C or gas mark 6 for 30 minutes or until slightly brown.
5 Serve hot or cold, in mounds, topped with fromage frais and surrounded by fruit.

BRAIN HERB

SAGE

It's no accident that the name of this herb is also used to denote a wise person, judgement or decision. Although its botanical name, *Salvia officinalis*, comes from the Latin, meaning 'healing plant', it is now known that sage has very specific beneficial effects on the memory – making it a perfect brain food. Not for nothing does the old proverb ask, 'How can a man grow old if he has sage in his garden?'

There are around 700 varieties of sage. Although native to Mediterranean countries, it is now cultivated throughout the world. It's a simple herb to grow in the garden or in a large pot on a terrace, and will easily survive a British winter, except when conditions are particularly harsh.

In the UK, sage is traditionally used as one of the main ingredients of stuffings for joints of meat. This is because, among its other therapeutic effects, it stimulates the production of bile, the digestive fluid secreted from the liver which encourages the digestion of fats. Of course, it has other culinary uses, too, as the recipes in this chapter have shown.

Sage is also used in herbal medicine as an antiseptic (rub a few leaves on bites and stings to relieve the tingling) and as an anti-inflammatory: gargling with sage tea eases the pain of gum infections, mouth ulcers and sore throats.

Yet that is not the end of sage's many medicinal qualities. Thanks to its high content of thujone, a phytoestrogen ('phyto' means 'plant'), it can help with menstrual problems and ease the discomfort of hot flushes in menopausal women. Herbalists also suggest using it to treat chest infections.

BRAIN SPICE

CHILLI

Although chillies are relatively new to this country, they've been grown in Central and South America for around 7,000 years. They have now been adopted by many of the world's leading cuisines, from West Indian to Turkish and Indonesian. In fact, they're one of the most widely grown spices in the world.

Chillies are members of the capsicum, or pepper, family, and there are hundreds of different varieties, from the fiery hot cayenne to the slightly milder dried chillies that are so popular in Spanish food. Apart from the less intense green peppers, they are not easy to grow in this country, but many are now sold fresh in most supermarkets — and, of course, they also come dried and powdered as packaged spices.

As you can probably guess from their strong, hot flavour, chillies are a powerful stimulant. Their main active ingredient, capsaicin, helps increase blood flow — including circulation to the brain, which makes them good brain food — and keeps the nervous system healthy. Chillies encourage a good appetite and soothe indigestion, and they're antibacterial and useful for easing colds and sore throats. Its fiery sensation notwithstanding, capsaicin is also believed to protect the stomach by increasing blood flow to its lining.

Most people know chilli best as the 'heat factor' in dishes such as chilli con carne. Used with care, however, it can also add flavour to milder dishes such as the Easy Cheese Frittata (page 34). Even so, it's best to follow a few safety precautions whenever you cook with chillies. Always remove the hot seeds before cooking with chillies; wash your hands well after chopping the fruit; wear gloves if you've got any cuts or abrasions on your hands; and don't, whatever you do, rub your eyes until all traces of chilli are gone.

SNOOZE FOODS

z z Z z

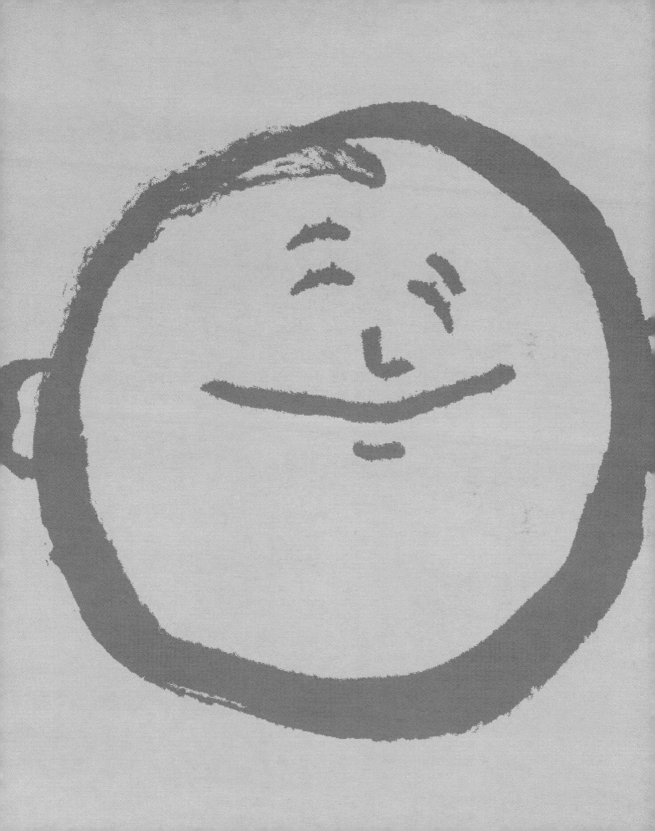

SNOOZE FOODS

Few people get through life without the occasional sleepless night, yet the odd loss of beauty sleep isn't a problem. Sadly, however, there is a huge army of people whose lives are plagued by chronic insomnia. Despite the fact that this is hardly a terminal disease, it can become an obsessive problem and often destroys people's quality of life.

There are many underlying causes of poor sleep, and habitual insomnia needs to be thoroughly investigated and treated appropriately. Limping through life on the crutch of sleeping pills isn't the answer, and there is no doubt that food can be a major factor in both the cause and relief of this miserable condition. No one, for instance, will sleep peacefully two hours after a huge bowl of chicken vindaloo and three pints of lager. Nor will you drift into the land of nod if you go to bed hungry. The first step, then, is to eat appropriate amounts of food at appropriate times. Secondly, it's vital to make use of all the herbs, spices and specific foods which help encourage calmness, relaxation and somnolence.

Herbal teas are a simple and effective starting point, and some are equally appropriate for children as well as adults. In southern Europe, weak chamomile tea sweetened with honey is a common remedy for fractious children, especially if they have a slight headache, a raised temperature and are very restless. Lime blossom is an excellent calmative for adults and makes a delicious tea, which is as nice to drink as it is effective. Valerian, hops, passion-flower and lavender are also valuable sleep aids, and can be used as fresh or dried herbs, essential oils, liquid extracts or tablets. They can be used in cooking, added to the bath, placed in a room fragrancer or used as massage oils. Culinary herbs are all fine during pregnancy and breastfeeding, but check with a pharmacist, herbalist or properly qualified aromatherapist before using them as essential oils or medicines, as some are best avoided at these times.

The dishes in this chapter are not only great to eat and not in the least 'medicinal', but they will also dispatch you into the arms of Morpheus, the god of sleep, without having to count a single sheep. Milk features in a number of these recipes, as it is one of the traditional foods that trigger the release of brain-calming tryptophans. The same is true of most starchy foods – which is why many of the commercial bedtime drinks that combine milk with malted barley and other cereals are so effective.

When they had sleep problems, the ancient Greeks used the sticky sap extracted from wild lettuce. The reason? It contains chemicals that are similar to morphine – which makes lettuce a powerful sleep-inducer. All modern lettuces are descended from the wild lettuce, and although they contain much smaller amounts of this active ingredient, they're fabulous sleep aids and crop up in a number of recipes. A bedtime lettuce sandwich is a perfect combination of natural sleep-inducing substances and starch; it will get you to sleep, it's not addictive like sleeping pills and you'll wake up without feeling the 'drug hangover' that so often accompanies pills.

Turkey, oily fish, green vegetables, bananas and nutmeg are among the other ingredients that will help you achieve a better night's sleep. Any recipes that include a couple of these should be on your regular menu if you find yourself staring at the ceiling on a frequent basis.

A good nightcap for the insomniac is the traditional cup of hot cocoa – and the good news is that chocolate in any form is a good prescription for the sleepless. Although chocolate does contain caffeine, this stimulant is present only in very small amounts. As long as you don't over-indulge, the mood-changing and soporific effects of its other main ingredient, theobromine, far outweigh the stimulating action of the caffeine. So take heart: you *can* eat your way to a better night's sleep – and sweeter dreams.

SUPER SNOOZER

All modern lettuces are descended from the original wild lettuce used by the ancient Greeks to make sleeping draughts. The sap contains a plant chemical that has an action similar to mild opiates. Though modern lettuces aren't as potent as the wild variety, a glass of this juice will still make counting sheep redundant. The mild hallucinogenic effects of the nutmeg also guarantee sweet dreams.

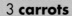

3 **carrots**
2 juicy **English apples**, such as Cox, Bramley, Russet, etc
½ a **cos lettuce**
a sprinkle of **nutmeg**

1 Run the first three ingredients through a juicer.
2 Pour in a glass, sprinkle with nutmeg and serve.

CHEF'S NOTE: Don't be tempted to use any other lettuce than cos for this recipe. It's rich in betacarotene, has a stronger flavour and contains more of the snooze-power chemicals than the paler green varieties such as little gems or iceberg.

LULLABY LETTUCE SOUP

If you go to bed every night praying to be carried off to the land of nod, this delicious soup will provide the answer. The B vitamins and enzymes in the chicken stock will calm your nerves, and the extraordinary chemicals in the lettuce will bring you hours of refreshing sleep. Lettuce seeds have been found in the most ancient Egyptian tombs; no doubt the pharoahs rest well in the afterlife!

1 medium **onion**, chopped
½ a **garlic** clove, chopped
4 tbsps **extra-virgin olive oil**
1.2 litres or 40fl oz light **chicken stock**
6 **lettuce hearts**, thoroughly washed and shredded
225ml or 8fl oz plain **bio-yoghurt**
a handful of **chives**, finely snipped

1 In a large saucepan, soften the onion and garlic in the oil.
2 Add the chicken stock and bring to a boil.
3 Stir in the lettuce and simmer gently for 10 minutes.
4 Stir in the yoghurt.
5 Serve hot or cold, sprinkled with chives as a garnish.

CAULI-BROCCI CHEESE

Cheese doesn't bring on nightmares. In fact, it's the tryptophan in cheese that stimulates the brain's production of relaxing hormones and helps induce sleep. The nightmare myth was spread by Victorian men when The Temperance Society tried to stop them drinking. Husbands put the blame for their restless nights on the Stilton, when in fact over-consumption of port was the real cause.

25g or 1oz **unsalted butter**
2 tbsps **white flour**
250ml or 9fl oz **milk**
140g or 5oz mature **organic Cheddar cheese**, grated
1 small **cauliflower**, in florets, blanched for 8 minutes
1 medium head of **broccoli** florets, blanched for 4 minutes
a handful of **pumpkin seeds**, husks removed
1 **beef tomato**, finely sliced

1 In a large saucepan, melt the butter gently. Mix in the flour and cook, stirring constantly, for three minutes.

2 Still stirring, add the milk gradually until a smooth cream develops.

3 Add three-quarters of the cheese and mix until melted.

4 Arrange the cauliflower and broccoli alternately in a shallow oven-proof dish and pour over the cheese sauce.

5 Sprinkle over with the pumpkin seeds. Arrange the tomato slices on top and sprinkle with the remaining cheese.

6 Bake at 220°C or 425°F or gas mark 7 for 15 minutes, until the cheese bubbles.

DREAM-TIME RISOTTO

Artichokes contain the chemical cynarin, which stimulates the liver and improves the general digestion of fats. By combining these often ignored vegetables with the sleep-inducing benefits of rice, the mind-calming borneol of basil and the relaxing citronella found in lemon balm, this recipe is quick, easy and a perfect dish to serve as a prelude to a sound night's sleep.

1 **garlic** clove, finely chopped
55g or 2oz **unsalted butter**
450g or 1lb can **artichoke hearts**, drained, rinsed and quartered
850ml or 29fl oz **organic vegetable stock**
225g or 8oz **arborio rice**
½ a handful of **fresh basil**, chopped
½ a handful of **lemon balm**, chopped
85g or 3oz mild **dolcellate cheese**, crumbled

1 In a large saucepan, soften the garlic in half the butter. Add the artichoke hearts and enough of the stock to cover. Simmer gently until tender – approximatley 10 to 15 minutes.
2 Mix in the rice and add the rest of the stock gradually, as it's absorbed, stirring constantly – approximately 15 to 20 minutes.
3 When the rice is almost cooked, stir in half of the dolcellate and most of the herbs.
4 Sprinkle the rest of the cheese and herbs on top – and serve.

HUSHABY HERRINGS

Herrings are rich in omega-3 and omega-6 fatty acids, which soothe joint and muscle pains with their anti-inflammatory properties. Oats are a rich source of B vitamins. Like all complex carbohydrates, oats stimulate the release of brain-calming tryptophan. Add the fenchone from dill or fennel, and you have a recipe for happy, sleep-filled nights.

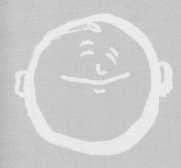

1 **onion**, chopped finely
55g or 2oz butter
85g or 3oz **baby spinach leaves**, roughly torn
40g or 1½ oz **Red Leicester cheese**, grated
140g or 5oz **oatmeal**
2 **herrings**, cleaned and gutted
2 **eggs**
3 tbsps **dill** or **fennel leaves**, finely chopped

1 In a small saucepan or skillet, soften the onion in the butter. Stir in the spinach and cook for two minutes.

2 Remove from heat. Add the cheese, 25g or 1oz of the oatmeal and season to taste.

3 Place the mixture inside the fish cavities and tie up with fine string.

4 Beat the eggs. Mix the remaining oatmeal with the dill or fennel leaves.

5 Roll each herring first in the beaten egg, then in the rest of the oatmeal and herb mixture.

6 Grill the herrings, under a pre-heated medium heat, for about eight minutes each side.

SLEEPY SESAME CHICKEN

The combination of B vitamins in chicken and vitamin E from the sesame seeds ensures a calm nervous system and good circulation. In addition, sesame seeds are especially rich in niacin and folic acid. This light, easily digested recipe makes a quick and perfect meal after a busy day. Indigestion is a common cause of insomnia, but you won't suffer after eating this dish.

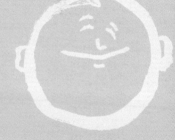

6 tbsps **sesame oil**
1 boneless, skinless **chicken breast**, cut into very slim goujons
1 **garlic** clove, finely chopped
1 tsp **sesame seeds**
350g or 12oz **mixed vegetables**: carrots, celery, courgettes, beans, peppers, cut into julienne strips
200ml or 7fl oz **organic vegetable stock**
85g or 3oz trimmed **asparagus spears**
225g or 8oz can **crushed tomatoes**

1 Heat the sesame oil in a wok or large saucepan.
2 Stir-fry the chicken, garlic and sesame seeds for five minutes.
3 Add the mixed vegetables and continue cooking for another five to seven minutes.
4 Stir in the tomatoes, stock and asparagus spears and simmer until the vegetables are tender – approximately five to ten minutes.
5 Serve with rice.

TANGY TURKEY

Turkey, like chicken, is rich in nerve-soothing and sleep-inducing B vitamins and enzymes. The marjoram in this recipe provides sabinene and eugenol – volatile oils which improve digestion and encourage relaxation. The addition of the rice wine is yet another aid to good sleep – but be careful with alcohol, as too much deprives you of dream sequences and you end up waking feeling unrefreshed.

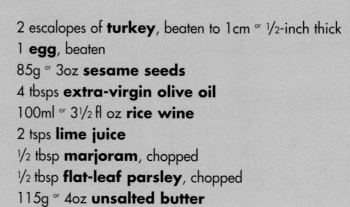

2 escalopes of **turkey**, beaten to 1cm ^{or} ½-inch thick
1 **egg**, beaten
85g ^{or} 3oz **sesame seeds**
4 tbsps **extra-virgin olive oil**
100ml ^{or} 3½ fl oz **rice wine**
2 tsps **lime juice**
½ tbsp **marjoram**, chopped
½ tbsp **flat-leaf parsley**, chopped
115g ^{or} 4oz **unsalted butter**

1 Dip the escalopes in the beaten egg, then in the sesame seeds, pressing the seeds in firmly.
2 In a large skillet, fry the escalopes in hot oil for three minutes each side. Remove and keep warm.
3 Add the wine to the skillet and boil for five minutes. Add the lime juice and herbs.
4 Lower the heat; whisk in the butter until the sauce is golden and glazed.
5 Pour the sauce over the meat and serve with noodles.

LIVER DE LA NUIT

Two of the most common causes of disturbed sleep are cramp and restless legs. Although the combination of liver and black pudding sounds rich and heavy, this is in fact a light and digestible dish. It is overflowing with vitamin A and iron, with the added benefit of potassium from the apples. The iron helps avoid restless legs, while the potassium helps prevent cramp.

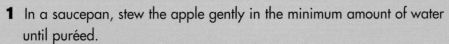

1 large **Bramley apple**
55g or 2oz **black pudding**
1 small **onion**, finely sliced
2 tbsps **extra-virgin olive oil**
55g or 2oz **unsalted butter**
4 thin slices of **organic calves' liver**,
about 115g or 4oz each

1 In a saucepan, stew the apple gently in the minimum amount of water until puréed.
2 In a non-stick pan, fry the black pudding gently until soft, but not crisp; then crumble it into the apple purée and keep warm.
4 In a large frying pan, cook the onion in the oil and butter to amost crisp.
5 Add the liver slices and cook for one minute each side.
6 To serve, spread the apple purée on warm plates, then place the liver in the middle and pile the onions around the side.

CHEF'S NOTE: Buy organic liver if you can, as this organ stores toxic residues from pesticides, herbicides, insecticides and growth hormones.

DDG CHOCOLATE CREPES

'DDG' stands for 'drop-dead gorgeous'. One taste, and you'll understand why.Chocolate, alcohol, Cape gooseberries and pancakes – is there a better recipe for heaven on a plate? Theobromine in the chocolate and the liqueur are both soothing and relaxing. And what a great way of getting sleep-inducing tryptophan from milk!

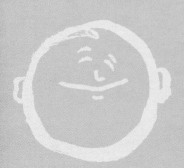

90g or 3¼ oz **plain flour**
15g or ½ oz **cocoa powder**
1 **egg**, beaten
200ml or 7fl oz **milk**
2 tbsps **butter**
4 tbsps **Kahlua** or **Tia Maria**
1 punnet of **Cape gooseberries**

1 Beat the flour, cocoa powder, egg and milk together until completely blended. Heat half the butter in a shallow frying pan.
2 Add a ladleful of batter to the pan; cook until golden – approximately three minutes. Flip and cook the other side for three minutes.
3 Continue with the rest of the batter until you have six or eight crêpes.
4 Drizzle Kahlua or Tia Maria liqueur on the top, surround with Cape gooseberries and serve.

CHEF'S NOTE: Cape gooseberries (botanical name Physalis) are usually served as petits fours dipped in sweet, sticky fondant icing. What a waste! They're delicious, tangy fruits, which complement the powerful flavours of these chocolate pancakes.

BEDTIME TEA-BREAD

This is the perfect accompaniment to your bedtime cuppa – lots of good starch to relax the mind, the natural sugar and iron in dates to nourish the blood and the wonderful soporific properties of lime blossom. Throughout Europe, lime-blossom tea is a traditional remedy for insomnia in both children and adults. This tea-bread will help people of all ages enjoy a good night's sleep.

5 **lime-blossom tea bags**
300ml or 10fl oz **boiling water**
450g or 1lb stoned **dried dates**, chopped
200g or 7oz **soft brown sugar**
1 **egg**, beaten
250g or 9oz **organic self-raising flour**

1 Soak the tea bags in the boiling water. Leave until cold. Squeeze the tea bags into the tea and discard.
2 Mix the tea thoroughly with all the other ingredients and leave to rest for at least six hours.
3 Line a 1.2-litre or 2-pint loaf tin neatly with greaseproof paper.
4 Pour the mixture into the tin and bake for 30 minutes at 180°C or 350°F or gas mark 4. Cool and serve.

SNOOZE HERB

LIME BLOSSOM

It has to be said that this gorgeous herb doesn't have the most politically correct provenance. Greek folklore traces it back to the rape of a nymph called Philyra by the god Saturn. She then gave birth to Chiron, a centaur, born with the upper body of a man and the legs of a horse.

Understandably, Philyra wasn't best pleased: after all, her son had no chance of winning a baby-of-the-year competition. In fact, she was so devastated that she asked the other gods not to allow her to continue living as human being, but to turn her into a lime tree. (Well, you would, wouldn't you?) What Philyra didn't know was that, thousands of years later, lime blossom would become one of the most exquisite, subtle, but sadly, little-known herbs in the Western world.

Tiliacea, to give lime its proper name, contains, among other wonderfully beneficial components, flavonoids which improve circulation, and compounds similar to benzodiazepene, the prescription tranquillizer, which many studies have found to be addictive. In lime blossom, however, these chemicals are natural, which makes it a wonderful non-addictive sedative and tension-reliever. It can also ward off panic attacks and palpitations – which makes it a brilliant snooze herb. In addition, it is used by herbalists to soothe headaches, particularly when caused by sinus problems.

The herbal remedy lime blossom isn't related to the citrus-fruit lime. And although it's not easy to find in your local supermarket, loose lime blossom or lime-blossom tea bags are available in most healthfood stores. It can be used to add extra flavour to stock, soups – or, as you can see on page 57 – as a brilliant addition to tea-breads.

SNOOZE SPICE

NUTMEG

If you've ever noticed a similarity between nutmeg and mace, it's not surprising. They both come from the same tree, *Myristica fragrans*, a large, long-living evergreen which grows abundantly in the Spice Islands. The British were, in part, responsible for the wide-scale cultivation of *Myristica fragrans*. They founded large plantations in the Far East during the 18th century, and also introduced the tree to the West Indies, which now produce a large proportion of world supplies.

In Britain, both nutmeg and mace are traditionally used in sweet dishes, particularly sprinkled on rice pudding or French toast and to flavour fruitcakes and Christmas puddings. Victorian nannies were especially fond of nutmeg – and for good reason. It contains myristicin and elemicin, which have a mildly soporific effect. A calming bowl of rice pudding might mean their young charges would settle down to sleep and nanny could have an evening off.

Other nationalities are more adventurous with these adaptable spices. Indians add them to dishes dating back to the mogul times of the 16th century. They're used in China, Asia and, particularly, the Middle East, where nutmeg is regarded as a traditional addition to many lamb recipes. No Dutch kitchen is complete without nutmeg (it's added to vegetable dishes, particularly mashed potato), and Italians give pasta an oriental flavour by sprinkling it over the finished dish. Both nutmeg and mace can be used – sparingly – to add an exotic touch to soups, sauces and stocks.

Nutmeg and mace are also used to treat chest problems and rheumatism, mainly in Eastern natural medicine; as well as to induce a sense of calm in troubled patients.

WAKE-UP FOODS

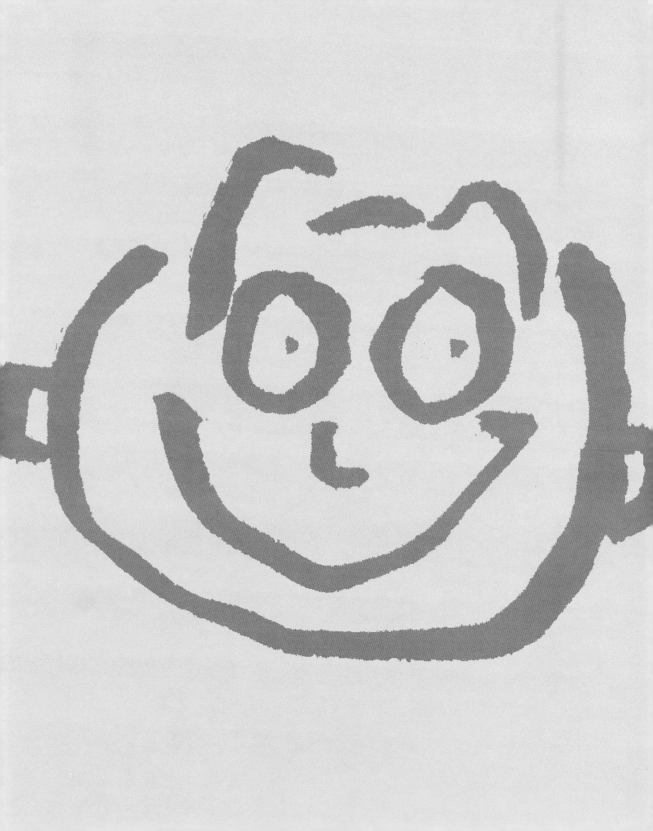

WAKE-UP FOODS

Tiredness is one of the most common reasons why people consult their doctors. Everyday, millions of people wake up feeling exhausted, lethargic and – as teenagers might say – totally knackered. They may be suffering some underlying illness such as anaemia, an underactive thyroid, glandular fever, ME, diabetes or that most depressing of all acronyms, TATT (Tired All The Time Syndrome).

While chronic exhaustion may well be caused by all of the above, not to mention insomnia, overwork, depression or the enormous burden of being a mother with young children, the truth is that the most commonly ignored reason for it – and often the simplest of remedies – is food. Constant dieting and foolhardy attempts to stick to ridiculously low-calorie diets, the over-consumption of energy-draining foods and eating disorders such as anorexia nervosa and bulimia can all deplete energy input – and not just in terms of calories, but also in terms of the essential nutrients your body needs in order to function at anything approaching its full potential.

Of course, the first step for anyone who is constantly tired must be a visit to the doctor in order to exclude all possible medical causes. Once you've got the all-clear, then it's time to try the wake-up recipes in this section, which will help restore you to vim, vigour and an active life. Of course, when you're feeling less than energetic, the last thing you want is to be faced with complex and difficult recipes – which is why all these wake-up recipes are simple to prepare.

There are some other points to consider when trying to implement a wide-awake diet. When many people feel exhausted, their first instinct is to reach for high-sugar items such as biscuits, sweets, chocolate and sweetened fizzy drinks, or to put loads of sugar in their tea. Unfortunately, these are the first steps on the sticky slope to the sugar trap, which you must avoid at all costs.

The reason? Your body produces huge amounts of insulin to deal with large amounts of sugar and convert it into energy. When you consume refined sugar, these chemical reactions happen very quickly. Once this sugar has been used up, the surplus insulin gets to work on your body's sugar reserves; before you know it, you've lurched from a state of high blood-sugar activity to low blood-sugar lethargy within the space of minutes. As the level of your blood sugar plummets, the craving for more sugar returns and the cycle repeats itself over and over again.

What you really need is an eating pattern that provides a combination of quick-release natural sugars from sweet fruits (fresh and dried), the slower-release sugars from more complex carbohydrates, such as bananas, potatoes, oats, pasta, rice and protein, and the slowest-release energy foods, like fish, meat, poultry, cheese and beans.

Your pattern of eating is also important. If you want to get up wide-awake and stay that way until bedtime, you need to become a 'grazer'. This means never going for more than three hours without a snack, which includes all three types of energy-releasing foods: fresh and dried fruits, complex carbohydrates and slow-release protein.

You'll find plenty of recipes for just this sort of eating plan in this chapter. Here, stimulating everyday foods such as apples, bananas, beetroot and fish rub shoulders with more exotic ingredients like cinnamon, turmeric, chervil, couscous and sunflower seeds. The section kicks off with an instant, energizing start to your day: a Wakey-Shakey smoothie (page 64) that will pop open your eyes and give you a wake-up call you probably haven't enjoyed for months. Work your way through the other recipes in this section, and you'll soon discover what it's like to have that lively feeling all day long.

WAKEY-SHAKEY

Apart from its nutritional benefits, the zingy flavour of cinnamon filters through peanut butter and yoghurt to form a wake-up call all on its own. Instant energy from the apples and pears, and slower-release energy from the bananas are enough to give anyone a kick-start in the morning. Add the powerful tonic effect of cinnamon's volatile oil cinnamaldehyde, and you've got a real clarion call.

2 **apples**, any variety apart from cooking apples
1 **pear**
2 **bananas**
1 tbsp **smooth peanut butter**
100ml or 3½ fl oz plain **bio-yoghurt**
½ tsp **cinnamon**

1 Run the first three ingredients through a juicer.
2 Pour the mixture into a bowl and beat in the peanut butter and yoghurt.
3 Pour into glasses, sprinkle cinnamon on top, and serve.

RED REVEILLE SOUP

If you're feeling sleepy and lethargic, here's a soup that will make sure you're wide-awake and full of wit even at the most demanding of dinner parties. You may not think it sounds like a breakfast dish, but if it's strained and chilled overnight, an early-morning glass provides a shot in the arm. The perfect marriage of beetroot and apples provides flavour and a cocktail of natural nutrients.

1 **onion**, finely chopped
3 tbsps **rape-seed** or **peanut oil**
3 small, uncooked **beetroots**, peeled and finely diced
2 **English apples**, peeled, cored and quartered
¼ **Savoy cabbage**, finely sliced
850ml or 29fl oz **organic vegetable stock**

1 Sweat the onion in the oil. Add the beetroot and soften gently for 20 minutes.
2 Mix in the apples, most of the cabbage and the stock.
3 Simmer, covered, until the vegetables are tender – about 25 minutes.
4 Stir in the reserved cabbage and serve.

SPICY SCRAMBLED EGGS

This unusual but tasty dish makes the perfect eye-opener for breakfast, lunch or supper. The unique flavour of turmeric and its action as an instant stimulator complements the high-protein content of the eggs, which provide long-term energy.

3 tbsps **butter**
1/2 tsp **turmeric**
2 small **courgettes**, grated
5 organic, free-range **eggs**, lightly beaten

1 In a saucepan, heat the butter and gently fry the turmeric for two minutes.
2 Stir in the courgettes and cook for one minute.
3 Add the beaten eggs and cook, folding occasionally, until lightly scrambled.

CHEF'S NOTE: Many people tend to over-scramble scrambled eggs. I think the best way to cook them is to leave the mixture until it starts to set, then, using a palette knife, begin to push it in gently from the sides so that you can still see the difference between the white and the yolks. Organic and free-range is the essential choice for a wide-awake dish, as this means there is virtually no risk of salmonella poisoning.

QUICK LORRAINE

It will take just one bite of this unusual quiche to get you buzzing. Lots of vitamin C, masses of betacarotene, all those friendly, active little 'bugs' in the yoghurt and the essential oil thymol in the thyme and marjoram will invigorate your taste buds and your sense of smell.

4 tbsps **extra-virgin olive oil**
1 small **onion**, thinly sliced
½ a **red** and **orange pepper**, deseeded and cut into small cubes
1 small **courgette**, thinly sliced
1 tbsp **dried marjoram**
1 tbsp **thyme**
2 **eggs**
225g or 8oz **mascarpone cheese**
25g or 1oz **Parmesan cheese**, grated
150ml or 5fl oz plain **bio-yoghurt**
1 sheet of ready-made **shortcrust pastry**, baked blind in a 25cm or 10-inch flan case for 15 minutes

1 In a frying pan, heat the oil and sweat the onion, peppers and courgette. Add the marjoram and thyme, and continue cooking gently for two minutes.

2 Beat the eggs. Then mix in the mascarpone, Parmesan and yoghurt.

3 Place the softened vegetables into the pastry case. Pour in the egg and cheese mixture. Bake at 200°C or 400°C or gas mark 6 for 30 minutes.

4 Serve with a fresh green salad.

PEP-UP PIZZA

If you've had a late night, an early start and a frantic morning, and all you feel like is a 20-minute nap at lunchtime, then this is the culinary answer that guarantees to keep you wide-awake in the afternoon.

450g or 1lb strong **white bread flour**
1 tsp **salt**
½ tsp **sugar**
6g or just over ⅛ oz **fast-action yeast**
75ml or 2½ fl oz **extra-virgin olive oil**
16 **basil leaves**
115g or 4oz soft **goats' cheese**, crumbled,
115g or 4oz **buffalo mozzarella**, finely diced

1 Blend the flour, salt, sugar and yeast in a food processor for 30 seconds, or mix thoroughly by hand.

2 Add three tablespoons of the oil, then 150ml or 5fl oz warm water and mix until the mixture looks like breadcrumbs.

3 Add another 150ml or 5fl oz warm water. Continue processing for three more minutes, or mix by hand until to a smooth, spongy dough.

4 Place the dough on a floured board and knead for two minutes. Brush it very lightly with olive oil, cover and let rise in a warm place for one hour. (An airing cupboard or barely warmed oven is ideal.)

5 Punch down the dough, divide it and roll or pat out into two thin, flat, round pieces. Transfer to a greased baking sheet. Brush with olive oil and arrange the basil leaves, then the cheeses, on top.

6 Bake at 220°C or 425°F or gas mark 7 for 12 minutes.

7 Serve with a fresh green salad.

CRUSTACEAN COUSCOUS

All shellfish make good wake-up meals, partly because they're light and easy to digest. When combined with the equally beneficial effects of the carbohydrate in couscous and the stimulating natural chemicals in chives, they will easily ward off any post-prandial somnolence.

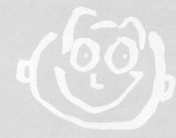

280g or 10oz **couscous**
8 **spring onions**, finely chopped
a handful of **chives**, finely snipped
½ a medium **cucumber**, peeled, deseeded and cut into julienne strips
8 **cherry tomatoes**, quartered
225g or 8oz cooked **shrimp**, shells removed
8 tbsps **vinaigrette dressing**
3 tbsps **lemon juice**

1 Wash the couscous thoroughly, then simmer in water for 20 minutes, stirring occasionally. Drain and allow to cool slightly.
2 Pour the couscous into a large bowl and add the next five ingredients. Mix thoroughly.
3 Stir in the vinaigrette, then the lemon juice.
4 Serve with warm wholemeal pitta bread.

A FISHY CAPER

If you want to be wide-awake enough for high-spirited pranks, then this is the dish for you. Chervil is not only rich in vitamin C, but also contains energizing coumarins. The capric acid in capers boosts the circulation, while essential fatty acids in salmon are good for the brain. What more do you need for a jolly caper?

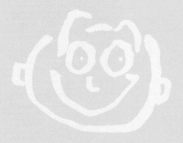

95ml or 3¼ fl oz **vegetable or fish stock**
3 sprigs of **chervil**
½ a **garlic** clove, well crushed
3 **spring onions**, finely chopped
315g or 11oz thick **salmon fillet**, skinned
2 tbsps **rape-seed oil**
2 plump **lettuce hearts**, cut into quarters and
    thoroughly washed
115g or 4oz **mange tout**, simmered for 5 minutes,
torn into chunks, drained, but kept warm
1 tbsp **capers**, soaked in **milk** for 5 minutes, then drained
1 **hard-boiled egg**, roughly chopped
95ml or 3¼ fl oz **vinaigrette dressing**

1 Warm the stock. Add the chervil, garlic and spring onions and set aside.
2 Brush the salmon with the oil. Grill for six minutes each side.
3 Arrange the lettuce and mange tout in a serving dish. Cut the salmon into chunks, place on top and sprinkle with the capers and the egg.
4 Mix the warm stock and vinaigrette together and pour over the salad.

CHICKEN PICK-ME-UP

When you need to be alert and wide-awake, there isn't a better combination than onions, chicken and the traditional herbs of the bouquet garni: sage, rosemary, thyme and chervil. They're all rich sources of volatile oils, which perk up the central nervous system and stimulate brain activity.

5 tbsps **extra-virgin olive oil**
1 **onion**, finely chopped
1 **garlic** clove, chopped
350g or 12oz **organic chicken breasts**, bonless,
skinless, cut into thin goujon slices
150ml or 5fl oz **organic vegetable stock**
55g or 2oz closed-cap **mushrooms**, sliced
55g or 2oz **green beans**, cut into 2.5cm or 1-inch batons
1 **bouquet garni**
125ml or 4fl oz **double cream**
125ml or 4fl oz plain **bio-yoghurt**

1 In a large skillet or saucepan, heat the oil and gently sweat the onion and garlic.
2 Add the chicken and stir-fry gently until golden brown.
3 Stir in the stock, mushrooms and beans. Add the bouquet garni.
4 Cover and continue cooking for about 15 minutes, until the chicken and vegetables are tender.
5 Pour off any excess liquid. Remove the bouquet garni. Stir in the double cream and yoghurt.
6 Serve with herb-flavoured rice or mashed potatoes.

TERRIFIC FRUITY TERRINE

Not an animal's liver in sight here: just the instant wake-up of tart lemon juice, energy-filled honey, sweet, succulent strawberries and the extra potassium in bananas. If you need to be awake for nocturnal activities, a late-night treat of this – with a modest glass of Champagne – is all you need.

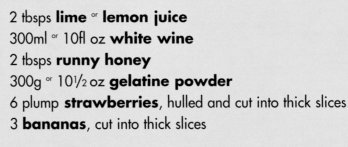

2 tbsps **lime** or **lemon juice**
300ml or 10fl oz **white wine**
2 tbsps **runny honey**
300g or 10½ oz **gelatine powder**
6 plump **strawberries**, hulled and cut into thick slices
3 **bananas**, cut into thick slices

1 Mix together the juice and the wine. Add the honey, stirring until it is dissolved.
2 Sprinkle the gelatine into four tablespoons of water until it swells in volume.
3 Line a 450g or 1lb cake tin with clingfilm and arrange the fruit inside.
4 Pour the gelatine mixture into a small, heat-proof container or saucepan and warm until it has completely dissolved.
5 Stir the gelatine into the wine mixture, then pour over the fruit.
6 Cover with clingfilm and chill until set.

PINE-A-BERRY COMPOTE

Whether served as a wonderful wake-up breakfast special or a perfect, energizing dessert, this mixture fits the bill. Stimulating enzymes and loads of energy-giving fruit sugar from the pineapple, the slightly tart flavour of the blueberries and the vitality minerals in nuts and seeds would wake up Rip van Winkle.

2 thick slices of fresh **pineapple**, cores removed
1 punnet of **blueberries**
115g or 4oz mixed crushed **seeds** and **nuts**
4 tbsps **runny honey**

1 Place the pineapple slices on an oven-proof plate.
2 Fill each core area with blueberries.
3 Scatter the seeds and nuts on top.
4 Drizzle with honey.
5 Place under a pre-heated hot grill for three minutes.

WAKE-UP HERB

CHERVIL

Despite the fact that it is one of the most ignored herbs, chervil is one of the most delicious and flexible of all culinary plants. You can add it to almost anything that specifies fines herbes, herb stock or a bouquet garni. It's easy to grow from seed and small enough for a pot on a windowsill or balcony, yet it costs a fortune to buy one of those small, plastic supermarket containers that last just a few days. And that's only if you can find it.

To me, growing chervil is one of the true delights of summer. Those small, bright-green leaves look as if they were created just to smile at a warm (but not too hot) sun. Within days of picking out a few sprigs to use in the kitchen, the plant is pushing up strong new stalks again.

Chervil – *Anthriscus cerefolium*, part of the *Umbelliferae* family – comes originally from the Middle East and southern Russia, where for centuries it has given its distinctive, slightly aniseed flavour to some of the cultures' traditional dishes. It's great in any herb combination, sprinkled over vegetables, in soups, salads and sauces and, as you can see on page 70, it also goes perfectly with fish.

Yet chervil does more than just taste good. It is a rich source of coumarins, flavonoids and volatile oil, which means it's a good general tonic – perfect when you're in need of a boost. It also helps purify the blood, provides useful amounts of iron, encourages good digestion and lowers high blood pressure. When sown in regular batches throughout the summer, it will keep you in fresh, healthy, wake-you-up leaves for the entire year.

WAKE-UP SPICE

TURMERIC

Marco Polo was one of the first Westerners to spot the potential of this mildly flavoured and useful herb. He said it reminded him of saffron. Little did he know that, in countries where saffron can be very expensive, many people do use turmeric in much the same way as saffron: to add a warm, yellow colour and pungent, bitter fragrance to white rice.

For centuries, however, the people of the East kept this spice a secret. In India, it was first used as a fabric dye, and today it forms one of the ingredients of a beauty paste. On some Pacific islands, chunks of the underground root are still worn as magic charms to fend off evil spirits.

It's in cooking, however, that turmeric enjoys its greatest success. It is included in practically every commercial curry paste and powder, and forms part of a wide range of Indian vegetarian food. In the West, many of our most popular processed foods include turmeric as a fragrant seasoning, along with a hint of pepper and ginger. It is also added to some mustard powders to give them that strong, pungent flavour.

Like all pungent spices, turmeric has a gentle, stimulating effect which is perfect if you arrive home after a busy day but can't just flop in front of the television. Many Eastern nations make full use of this, and take it as a general tonic. It is also used in Asia to ease liver problems.

Like most spices, turmeric doesn't need to be saved for hot dishes designed to give your taste buds a hefty kick. On page 66, for example, you can find an idea for a new look at scrambled eggs. Used sparingly, turmeric gives this breakfast or light supper dish a subtle taste of the Raj.

SEXY FOODS

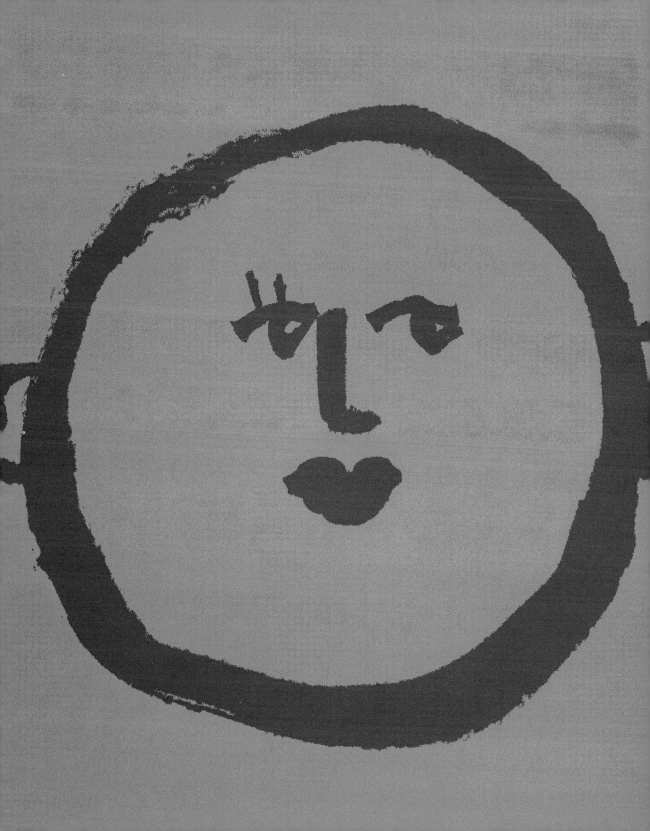

SEXY FOODS

Beauty, of course, is in the eye of the beholder, but the beauty of sexual attraction is far more than skin deep. Naturally, sexual attraction is a prerequisite for aphrodisia. But in the same way that make-up, hair styles, clothes and perfume can set the seal on a romantic encounter, food, too, can add its special magic.

Most everyone knows that there is no such thing as a love potion. Yet, all things being equal, the right food in the right situation at the right time can heighten awareness, promote sensuality and act as the catalyst that turns the lead of friendship into the gold of passion.

Many foods have legendary aphrodisiac qualities – and there is often an element of truth in many of the recommendations of folklore and folk medicine. At the end of the day, however, whether the effect is real or imagined isn't important – it is the end result that counts. If you believe the legends and you eat the food, then you're highly likely to reap some rewards. That said, in this chapter you'll find recipes to suit every palate and any romantic situation. And they include foods that have not only stood the test of time, but have established a place within with the belief systems of widely differing cultures throughout the world.

Many of these romance foods do have scientifically proven benefits. Some improve the circulation, which is essential for both male performance and female enjoyment. Others induce emotional states of well-being and happiness; and they contain nutrients that are essential for physical activity, hormonal functions and general vital health.

Vitamin E, for example, a key ingredient for the sexual performance and enjoyment of both sexes, is found in avocados, nuts and seeds. You'll get iodine from the fish dishes in this section – and iodine is vital for the thyroid since, without it, this gland, which controls so many bodily functions, just won't work to its optimum capacity. It isn't coincidence, either, that eggs are one of the universal symbols of fertility, for they provide the nutrients needed in order to achieve it.

Tropical fruits such as mangoes, pawpaws and pineapples aren't only sensuous to eat, they are also rich in aphrodisiac enzymes. And as well as the performance-enhancing potassium in bananas, who can miss the obvious erotic symbolism of this remarkable fruit? You'll find recipes for oily fish, poultry and shellfish, all of which can play their part as delicious components of an amorous feast. The addition of traditional aphrodisiac herbs and spices such as coriander and ginger add the final touches to any romantic meal.

Of course, amorous eating must appeal to all the senses if it is going to succeed. For the optimum romantic enjoyment, food has to look good, smell good and taste good – just like your favourite lover. Ideally, the perfect romantic setting would be a beautiful tablecloth, fine crystal, elegant crockery and the finest cutlery combined with flattering candlelight and soft music. Every recipe in this section would be the ideal companion for such surroundings, but it's worth remembering that if the chemistry's right, fish and chips in a paper bag can also end in consuming passion. And while many of the other recipes in this book are designed to serve four people, every one in this chapter is strictly à deux.

PASSION PARLOUR

The expression 'to ginger someone up' means just what it says: the volatile oil gingerol in ginger is a powerful stimulant to the circulation. So, for obvious reasons, this wonderful spice has a long history in folklore as an aphrodisiac. Add the passion-fruit and garlic, and you have a unique blend of liquid erotica. For more mature lovers, celery will help cope with the occasional creaky joint.

4 thick, juicy **celery sticks**, well washed
½ a **garlic** clove
3 **passion-fruit**, outer shells removed
400g or 14oz **radicchio leaves**, thoroughly washed
2 pinches of ground **ginger**

1 Run the first the first four ingredients through a juicer.
2 Pour into two glasses, sprinkle with ginger and serve.

MANGAVO

This soup is specifically designed to be a shared loving cup. Avocados are a huge source of vitamin E, an essential nutrient for a sparkling love life. The beetroot not only colours this soup a romantic pink, but is a renowned blood tonic. The final touch is the delicate flavour of coriander, known throughout Asia as a gentle and long-acting aphrodisiac.

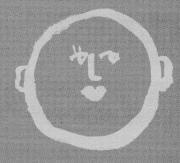

1 large organic **Hass avocado**, stone and skin removed, cut into chunks
1 large **organic mango**, stone and skin removed, cut into chunks
250ml or 9fl oz organic **beetroot juice**
200ml or 7fl oz plain **bio-yoghurt**
2 tbsps **coriander leaves**, finely chopped

1 Blend the first four ingredients in a food processor or blender.
2 Pour into a saucepan and heat just to the simmering point.
3 Serve in bowls, with a sprinkling of chopped coriander.

FLIRTY FLAN

Asparagus, the favourite of all European fantasy foods, is one example of truth residing in folklore. Extremely rich in potassium, folic acid and the natural plant chemical asparagine, asparagus is a particularly good romantic food-booster for men. The increased blood flow from cayenne and the vitamin E from sesame seeds are simply the amorous icing on the cake.

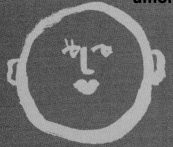

1 sheet of ready-made **puff pastry**
20 to 24 **asparagus tips**
2 small **eggs**
200ml or 7fl oz **organic fromage frais**
½ tsp **cayenne pepper**
1 tbsp **sesame seeds**

1 Use the pastry to line a greased 20cm or 8-inch flan tin.
2 Arrange the asparagus in a cartwheel design, with the green tips facing the rim.
3 Beat the eggs into the fromage frais. Stir in the cayenne pepper.
4 Pour the mixture over the asparagus tips. Sprinkle with sesame seeds.
5 Bake at 220°C or 425°F or gas mark 7 for 25 minutes.

MUSSEL POWER

All shellfish are known for their aphrodisiac properties – mainly because they are super-rich in the mineral zinc, which is vital for male sexuality. This is such a simple dish and incredibly easy to prepare. For maximum effect, serve it in one large bowl and share the sensuous pleasure of feeding each other with these little molluscs straight out of their shells.

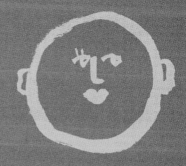

2kg or 4½lbs **mussels**, washed and scraped
25g or 1oz **unsalted butter**
1 **garlic** clove, finely chopped
3 **spring onions**, finely chopped
½ tsp **dried oregano**
1 glass of **dry white wine**
1 glass of **water**
4 tbsps **curly parsley**, finely chopped

1 Place the mussels in a large saucepan. Cover and heat until all the shells are open and the liquid inside them has drained out – approximately five minutes.

2 Strain the liquid through a piece of muslin and reserve.

3 Place the butter, garlic, spring onions and oregano in the saucepan and sweat gently for two minutes.

4 Add the reserved mussel liquor, the wine and the glass of water. Stir for another minute. Add the mussels, cover and boil briskly for five minutes.

5 Empty into a large bowl and sprinkle with parsley.

THREE-FISH CARPACCIO

The huge content of essential fatty acids in salmon and tuna are nature's gift to lovers, and the iodine in sea bass is a natural energy booster. Topped with the mood-enhancing essential oils in basil and washed down with a glass of pink Champagne, this is a fail-safe recipe for passion.

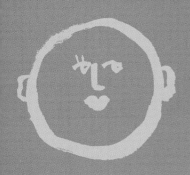

2 tsps **capers**
4 **lemons**
4 **limes**
6 tbsps best **extra-virgin olive oil**
3 tbsps **basil leaves**, roughly torn
6 sprigs of **dill**, stalks removed
1 x 225g or 8oz fillet *each* fresh **salmon**, **red tuna** and **sea bass**, all sliced paper-thin

1 Soak the drained capers in milk for 10 minutes, then drain and crush lightly in your fingers.
2 Juice three of the lemons and three of the limes.
3 Mix the oil, citrus juices, crushed capers, basil and dill.
4 Dip the fish pieces in the oil and herb mixture, place in a wide dish, cover and chill for at least six hours.
5 Serve garnished with wedges of the extra lemon and lime and chunky wholemeal bread.

CHEF'S NOTE: If you don't have an obliging fishmonger, here's an easy way to prepare the fish yourself. Just put the fillets in the freezer for 15 minutes and they'll slice perfectly with a long, sharp knife.

CHICKPEA TROUT

The great 20th-century songwriters captured the essence of the vital link between mood and love with songs such as 'I'm in the Mood for Love'. Loving mood food must create the same ambience. This light dish of heart-friendly trout, high-protein chickpeas and the pink from the chilli and paprika combine eye appeal with foods guaranteed to produce the perfect mood.

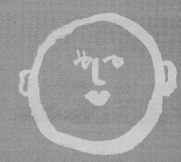

1 small **onion**, finely chopped
1 small **garlic** clove, finely chopped
4 tbsps **extra-virgin olive oil**
1 tsp **paprika**
1 tsp **chilli powder**
225g or 8oz can **chopped tomatoes**
400g or 14oz can **chickpeas**, thoroughly washed
4 pink **salmon trout** fillets
lemon slices
coriander leaves

1 In a saucepan or frying pan, sweat the onion and garlic in half the oil for five minutes.

2 Stir in the paprika and chilli powder and cook for two minutes.

3 Add the tomatoes and chickpeas and simmer until tender – about 10 minutes. Add more water if the mixture starts drying out. Mash the chickpeas roughly.

4 Pan-fry the trout fillets in the rest of the oil for two minutes each side.

5 To serve, place the chickpea mash on plates, top with the fish and garnish with lemon slices and coriander.

DRESSED BREAST

The romantic appeal of this dish lies in the starch in the rice, which encourages the release of mood-enhancing tryptophan from the brain, and in the pesto's high vitamin E content, which is so important for a healthy sex life. It makes another easy-to-prepare recipe that is also light and easy to digest.

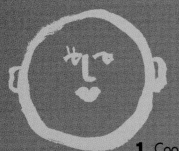

115g or 4oz **basmati rice**
1/2 a **green pepper**, deseeded and finely diced
3 **spring onions**, finely diced
55g or 2oz **unsalted butter**
4 tbsps **red pesto**, shop-bought or make your own
2 **organic chicken breasts**, boneless and skinless

1 Cook the rice according to the instructions, but add the pepper and spring onions halfway through the cooking time.
2 Mix the butter into the pesto and rub into each chicken breast. Reserve some leftover pesto mixture, being careful not to include any pesto that has been in contact with the uncooked chicken.
3 Grill the chicken pieces for eight to ten minutes on each side.
4 Spoon the rice onto plates and drizzle with surplus pesto mixture.
5 Place the chicken breasts on top to serve.

RARE, RICH & NUTTY

If red meat puts you in mind of red-blooded pursuits, then here's the perfect recipe. It's packed with iron, B vitamins and protein, and boasts an extra *frisson* from the spine-tingling Tabasco sauce. With the essential minerals in the walnuts and the slightly mysterious flavour of anchovies combined with steak, you won't need a starter and it will be hours before you get round to dessert.

115g or 4oz **chopped walnuts**
½ a **garlic** clove, finely chopped
½ can **anchovies**, drained, soaked in **milk** for 10 minutes and drained again
1 tsp **Tabasco sauce**
4 tbsps **peanut** or **rape-seed oil**
2 x 200g or 7oz **fillet steaks**, 1cm or ½-inch thick

1 Blend the walnuts, garlic, anchovies, Tabasco sauce and one tablespoon of the oil in a food processor.
2 Sear the steaks in the rest of the hot oil for 10 seconds each side.
3 Press the nut mixture into the steaks. Cover and chill for half an hour, then bake at 200°C or 400°C or gas mark 6 for 20 minutes.

AMOROUS BANANA SPLIT

This banana split is definitely for adults only. It's an X-rated dessert – and not because of the calories. Loads of potassium in the bananas prevents cramp at inappropriate moments, while the mysterious flavour of cardamom – widely regarded as an aphrodisiac in the Far East – and the heady aroma of sweet almonds from the Amaretto will transport you to images of a sultan's palace.

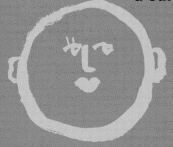

2 tsps ground **cardamom**
85ml or 3fl oz **orange juice**
50ml or 2fl oz **lemon juice**
2 tbsps **caster sugar**
3 tbsps **morello cherry jam**
25g or 1oz **butter**
4 **bananas**, peeled and split lengthways
3 tbsps **Amaretto**
4 tbsps flaked **almonds**

1 In a saucepan, warm the first six ingredients until well blended.
2 Place the bananas in an ovenproof dish so that they fit snugly.
3 Pour over the Amaretto, then the warm sauce.
4 Sprinkle with the flaked almonds and bake at 180°C or 350°F or gas mark 4 for 20 minutes.

BERRY GOOD SORBET

Granita, a popular romantic drink served at many cafés in Italy, is a bit like a half-frozen lemon sorbet. But add fresh raspberries, not only the most romantic of fruits but abundant in essential minerals, and the sweet crispness of langues du chat biscuits and you have a deliciously light dessert guaranteed to create that loving feeling. This dish is simply top of its class.

55g or 2oz **caster sugar**
350ml or 12fl oz **mineral water**
juice of 4 unwaxed **lemons**
1 punnet of **raspberries**
4 **langues du chat biscuits**

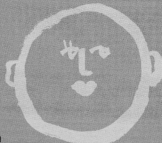

1 In a saucepan, gently dissolve the sugar in the water and lemon juice over a low heat. Cool.

2 Place the mixture in a freezer-proof container.

3 Freeze for two hours, breaking up the crystals every 30 minutes.

4 Place four raspberries in the bottom of two Champagne flutes or tall sundae dishes. Fill each with the granita mixture. Top with the rest of the fruit and serve with the biscuits on the side.

SEXY HERB

CORIANDER

Sprinkled over pasta, added to salad, mixed sparingly into scrambled eggs – and, as you'll have seen on page 81, stirred into soup – coriander is one of the 'sexy' herbs of the modern kitchen. You see it everywhere: used as a main ingredient in a salsa, on a salad in a top restaurant or as a topping on an inventive pizza. And of course, it's a basic part of Indian cuisine.

Coriander was cultivated in Egypt three centuries ago, and was so highly prized that it was placed in the tombs of Egyptian pharaohs. The Chinese believed it brought immortality – perhaps they borrowed this message from the Middle East, where it was also considered to be an aphrodisiac. (Did they expect to have a great sex life on the other side, I wonder?)

Whatever its surrounding myths, coriander does have real medicinal value.. It is a useful cleansing agent, and its volatile oils possess mood-enhancing properties which, combined with its flavonoids and phenolic acids, is thought to have some aphrodisiac effect. It is also good to use as a treatment for indigestion.

Coriander is easy to grow from seed – so easy, in fact, that you have to be careful how much you sow. Even in a cool British summer it will go from succulent young leaves to flowering within a week of continuous sun.

My dear friend Jekka McVicar, the UK's top herb grower, stakes up the long stems, allows the seeds to ripen, then dries them and adds them to soups, sauces and vegetable dishes. I must admit I can't be bothered. Instead, I put the flowers in salads and sow short rows of new seed about every two weeks so that I have a fresh supply of leaves all summer long.

SEXY SPICE

CAYENNE

Most of us know cayenne as simply a red pepper powder bought in jars or packets of spice, but cayenne is, in fact, a chilli – one of the hottest examples of the capsicum group of peppers. Like all members of this plant family, the cayenne pepper is rich in vitamin C, though, admittedly, not much is left in its dried form. Yet cayenne is still an all-round nutrient, particularly good at boosting immunity against colds, flu and other common ailments that we make such a fuss about in the West.

What many people don't realize is that it also helps digestion and is a good circulation-booster. This makes it extremely beneficial if you're planning a passionate night – it has been known to give long-term benefits to men's sexual prowess. Used as a medicine for many hundreds of years, its main ingredient is a naturally occurring chemical called capsaicin – and that is what gives cayenne its circulation-boosting properties.

Originally from South America, cayenne is now used around the world as a culinary spice and medicament. As with all the other peppers, it is the fruit of the plant that is used. Unlike many of its cousins, however, which tend to rot quite quickly, cayenne keeps well in a dry environment, and will maintain its pungent flavour in most kitchens for months on end.

Cayenne is a very flexible spice which can be used in curries, most Indian, Afro-Caribbean and Indonesian foods, and even mulled wines. It also gives extra punch to traditionally blander dishes such as scrambled eggs, savoury omelettes and practically anything made with minced beef or lamb, such as shepherd's or cottage pie or meatballs.

PEACE FOODS

Peace Foods

Stressed out after a hectic work week? Frazzled after a day of looking after boisterous children? Have the demands of modern living stretched your nerves so tight that you're just a few steps away from breaking point? Then take a deep breath, and take heart: this chapter contains all the foods you need to create moods of peace and tranquillity. The recipes listed in this section don't have the same effect as the snooze foods, which are designed specifically to help you sleep. Calm, peace and tranquillity are moods that everyone needs from time to time – even if they are certainly not the states of mind the majority of people enjoy in their day-to-day activities.

Yet that isn't necessarily a bad state of affairs. There are many misconceptions about stress and the role that it plays, especially in relation to conditions such as high blood pressure, stomach ulcers and headaches. Stress is part of the human natural survival mechanism, and is a direct response to the fight, fright and flight reflex. It is this stress response that puts the edge on performance, drives competitiveness and is a major contributor to success in our chosen endeavours. The recipes in this chapter aren't designed to insulate you from these beneficial effects of moderate levels of stress, but they will help you cope with periods of excessive stress in a positive way.

You'll find lots of good starches, such as wholemeal bread, rice, pasta and flour, in many of these suggestions. All of these are rich sources of B vitamins, which nourish the central nervous system and help the brain produce its wonderful peace-inducing tryptophans. Even the humble chicken liver, as it appears in Stressless Liver (page 101), becomes a multi-beneficial dish with the primary function of inducing peace and all the other nutritional benefits of iron, vitamin B12, vitamin C and fibre.

Herbs also play a major part in helping to bring a sense of calm into a hectic lifestyle. Rosemary, one of the most ancient of medicinal herbs, has many uses in areas involving both mood and mind function. Mint, especially when combined with wonderful dark, bitter chocolate, as it is in the Skinny Dip (page 105), is not only a delicious treat, but also induces almost instant feelings of peacefulness.

Since man's earliest times, many civilizations have used the extraordinary power of spices to alter mood. The Ayurvedic practitioners of India, the Chinese traditional herbalists, the amazingly knowledgeable Tibetan monks and the early inhabitants of the tropical Spice Islands all knew the value of these almost magical spices and used them widely in their food and medicine. Often, spices were included as an integral part of religious ceremonies in which inner peace and tranquillity were prime objectives. Garam masala, the spice mixture detailed on page 107, is just one example of the wide range of tropical spices that are renowned for their mood-altering medicinal values.

There are key times when these peace recipes will be of particularly good value. For example, how often, after a week of continual stress and effort, does your relaxing Sunday finish with a migraine? How many times have you struggled to clear your desk before going on holiday, packed your bags at 1AM, rushed to the airport, arrived at your destination – and become ill the next day? Experiences such as there aren't coincidental; in fact, they are your body's way of telling you that you've been pushing too hard and need to recharge your batteries. A few days of eating these dishes will help you unwind sufficiently to enjoy those delicious sensations of peacefulness which allow your immune system to get back to work and protect you from the everyday infections that attack all of us in times of stress.

PEACEFUL PUNCH

It wasn't just for flavour that Victorian nannies used to add nutmeg to rice pudding in the nursery. In tiny doses, myristicin, its mildly hallucinogenic compound, engenders feelings of peace and calm. With the aromatic substances in apples, the vitamin C and carotenoids in the kiwi fruit and the mildly soporific flavonoids in celery, a glass of this juice is better than any tranquillizer.

2 **apples**
4 **kiwi fruit**
1 **celery stick**, with leaves
1/2 tsp **nutmeg**

1 Run the first three ingredients through a juicer, reserving the celery leaves.
2 Dip the celery leaves in the nutmeg.
3 Pour into glasses and serve with the celery leaves on top.

CHARD CHOWDER

Redolent of country kitchens and traditional cooking, hot soup is the ultimate comfort food, and this chowder will take you even closer to nirvana than most. The hormone-balancing plant chemicals in sage, the antioxidants in oregano (traditional ingredients in herbes de Provence) and the nerve-nourishing B vitamins from lentils turn this nourishing soup into a bowl of serenity.

1 medium **onion**, chopped
3 **garlic** cloves, finely chopped
4 tbsps **extra-virgin olive oil**
25g or 1oz **butter**
175g or 6oz tiny **green lentils**, thoroughly rinsed
½ tsp **herbes de Provence**
650g or 1lb 7oz **chard** or **spinach**, thoroughly washed and roughly torn

1 In a large saucepan, soften the onion and garlic in the oil and butter.
2 Add the lentils, herbs and 850ml or 29fl oz water.
3 Boil briskly for 10 minutes, then simmer for 25 minutes until the lentils are almost tender.
4 Add the chard or spinach and simmer for another 10 minutes.
5 Liquidize if you like, but this soup tastes great left just as it is.

CHEF'S NOTE: This recipe would work with any pulse, but remember that some need soaking overnight and boiling for longer.

TOFU TREAT

The legendary plant hormones in soya are what make tofu the perfect peace food. By evening out fluctuations of hormones, tofu helps to maintain a balanced equilibrium, combating any associated adrenalin rush of stress and anxiety. The calm-inducing carbohydrates and the traditionally soothing benefits of honey are all present in this perfect recipe for peace.

200g or 7oz **tofu**
30ml or 1fl oz **soy sauce**
30ml or 1fl oz **balsamic vinegar**
2 tbsps **walnut oil**
1 tbsp **crushed capers**
1 tbsp **runny honey**
1 pack of prepared **stir-fry vegetables**
4 tbsps **safflower oil**

1 Cut the tofu into bite-sized cubes. Mix together the next five ingredients and use half the mixture to coat the tofu.
2 In an oven-proof casserole dish, bake the tofu at 220°C or 425°F or gas mark 7 for 15 minutes, stirring occasionally.
3 In a large frying pan or wok, stir-fry the vegetables in the safflower oil for four minutes.
4 Add the tofu and the rest of the sauce. Turn down the heat and warm through.
5 Serve on rice, noodles or spaghetti.

PEACEMEAL

At the end of a long, stressful day, nothing could be better than sharing a glass of chilled white wine with your partner while you prepare this quick and easy dish which will set you up for an evening of peaceful relaxation. Oats (a traditional calming food), soothing calcium from the whitebait and the peace-inducing aromatic oils in basil all make this an ideal beginning to a starry, starry night.

> 450g or 1lb **whitebait**
> 175g or 6oz **fine oatmeal** seasoned with **salt**, **pepper** and 2 tsps **dried dill**
> **rape-seed oil** – enough to fill a deep frying pan to a depth of 1cm or ½ inch
> 20 **basil leaves**, finely torn
> 150ml or 5fl oz **mayonnaise**
> 1 **lemon**, quartered

1 Wash the whitebait, dry thoroughly and roll in the seasoned oatmeal.

2 In a large frying pan, heat the oil and fry the fish in batches until slightly crisp – around three to four minutes. Keep each batch warm as you fry the others.

3 Mix the basil into the mayonnaise; spoon into two small ramekins.

4 Serve the fish garnished with lemon wedges and with the herb mayonnaise for dipping.

CHEF'S NOTE: Re-using oil is positively unhealthy, so don't use a deep-fat fryer for whitebait. Use good oil once only, and cook the fish in batches.

TINKY'S TREAT

We have five cats, but only one really wants to be in the house. Nothing could be more peaceful than watching Tinky curled up in front of the fire – especially after she has had the leftovers of this delicious salmon dish. Yet again, it's the calming essential oils from the fish, along with the stress-busting carvone in dill and a hint of alcohol from the vermouth, that does the trick. Purrr!!

1 x 350g or 12oz **fillet of salmon**, cut into 1cm or ½-inch strips
4 tbsps **plain white flour**, seasoned with **black pepper, celery salt** and **mixed fines herbes**
2 tbsps **extra-virgin olive oil**
a few sprigs of **dill**
1 sherry glass of **dry white vermouth**

1 Coat all of the salmon completely in the seasoned flour.
2 In a large frying pan, fry the fish in the hot oil, along with the sprigs of dill – approximately five to six minutes.
3 Remove the salmon with a slotted spoon and place in a warm dish.
4 Take the pan off the heat. Add the vermouth. Return the pan to the heat and bubble to reduce for three minutes.
5 Pour the sauce over the salmon. Serve with puréed potatoes and baby broad beans.

STRESSLESS LIVER

Liver is a prime ingredient in any recipe designed to reduce stress and anxiety. It contains vast amounts of vitamin A to build immunity, which may be severely damaged by long-term stress, and substantial quantities of B vitamins to nurture the entire central nervous system. Cooked here with grapes, a storehouse of aromatic compounds, this is the perfect de-stress dish.

2 **spring onions**, very finely chopped
1 small **garlic** clove, very finely chopped
3 tbsps **extra-virgin olive oil**
175g or 6oz **chicken livers**, membranes removed and cut into large chunks
55g or 2oz **flour** seasoned with **salt, pepper** and 1 tsp **paprika**
115g or 4oz **white seedless grapes**, peeled and halved
4 slices **wholemeal baguette**, lightly toasted
1 small bunch of **parsley**, finely chopped

1 In a large frying pan, soften the spring onions and garlic in the oil.
2 Roll the liver pieces in the seasoned flour. Turn up the heat and cook for three minutes, stirring constantly, until seared.
3 Add about half a cup of almost boiling water and simmer for one minute, scraping the pan thoroughly.
4 Take off the heat and mix in the grapes. Leave to rest for one minute.
5 Serve on the lightly toasted bread, scattered with parsley.

MAORI CHICKEN

The huge amount of vitamin C and bioflavonoids in kiwi fruit make this a much more interesting and peace-enhancing variation on traditional coronation chicken. Garam masala gives it a bit more bite and contains a mixture of anti-stress spices. Rice provides enough bulk to make a complete picnic, lunch or supper dish and encourages the brain's production of peace-inducing tryptophans.

1 tbsp **garam masala**
300ml or 10fl oz **mayonnaise**
350g or 12oz cooked and shredded **chicken**
85g or 3oz cooked **rice**
1 small **red onion**, very finely chopped
2 tender **celery sticks**, very finely chopped
115g or 4oz diced **red, yellow** or **green pepper**
125ml or 4fl oz **vinaigrette dressing**
3 **kiwi fruit**, peeled and cut into chunks

1 Mix the garam masala into the mayonnaise. Set aside.
2 In a large bowl, combine the chicken, rice and salad ingredients, mix well, then add the vinaigrette. Leave to rest for at least an hour.
3 Mix the mayonnaise into the salad and gently fold in the kiwi fruit, being careful not to break them. Serve with crusty wholemeal bread.

LAID-BACK LAMB

The traditional combination of lamb and rosemary isn't accidental – rosemary aids the digestion of fat and makes it easier for gastric juices to cope with the meat. But there's a hidden bonus, as the borneol from the rosemary is a true bringer of peace and happiness. The anchovies in this dish are a good source of essential fatty acids, which help the emotional transition from agitation to peacefulness.

1 small shoulder, or half shoulder of **lamb**
55g or 2oz well-seasoned **flour**
55g or 2oz can **anchovies**, drained
6 to 10 small sprigs of **rosemary**

1 Wash the lamb, dry thoroughly, remove any excess fat and rub over with the seasoned flour.

2 Using a sharp knife, make incisions at equal distance all over the meat.

3 Into each hole, push one anchovy and a sprig of rosemary.

4 Preheat the oven to its hottest temperature. Put in the meat, then turn down immediately to 190°C or 375°F or gas mark 5.

5 Roast for 25 minutes per 450g or 1lb, plus 25 minutes extra. Allow to rest for 15 minutes, covered with foil, before carving. Serve with your favourite vegetables.

PEACEFUL PRUNE PUD

The additional benefits of prunes – or any other dried fruit – make this a soothing dessert for the end of the day. The high natural sugar content of dried fruit keeps the blood-sugar supply to the brain on an even keel, which is emotionally relaxing. Tryptophan in the cheese and the lethargy-fighting components of cinnamon turn this into the most peaceful sweet around.

100g or 3½ oz **pudding rice**
1 tsp **lemon juice**
40g or 1½ oz **caster sugar**
700ml or 24fl oz **milk**
115g or 4oz **stoned prunes**, snipped
1 tsp **cinnamon**
2 tbsps **mascarpone cheese**

1 Place the rice, lemon juice and sugar in a large saucepan. Add about 200ml or 7fl oz water and simmer until the water is nearly absorbed.
2 Pour in the milk, and simmer for 10 minutes.
3 Add the prunes and continue simmering for 20 minutes, stirring occasionally, until rich and creamy.
4 Sprinkle with cinnamon and serve with a dollop of mascarpone.

SKINNY DIP

Of all the peaceful foods, none can compare with smooth, dark chocolate. Theobromine from cocoa beans generates feelings of peace and romance. Add the calming influence of mint and a little alcohol from the Kahlua, and you can enjoy all the benefits and flavours without any of the guilt. What's more, you'll get at least two of your five daily portions of fresh fruit from this delicious dessert.

85g or 3oz **dark chocolate**
125ml or 4fl oz **strong mint tea**
30ml or 1fl oz plain **bio-yoghurt**
25g or 1oz **butter**
3 tbsps **Kahlua**
115g or 4oz each **Cape gooseberries**,
cherries with stalks, **strawberries**, hulls attached,
preferably with stalks

1 In a saucepan, melt the chocolate into the mint tea over a very low heat.
2 Bring to the boil for one minute, then stir in the yoghurt.
3 Remove the pan from the heat, then stir in the butter and the liqueur.
4 Pour the sauce into a fondue pan, or place the saucepan over a night-light burner.
5 Serve the fruit on plates, and use forks to dip pieces into the chocolate sauce.

PEACE HERB

BASIL

In many minds, basil may be associated only with mozzarella, avocados and delicious Mediterranean nibbles squashed on earthy, crusty bread. In fact, it comes from India, and was also grown in the Middle East. Folklore has it that basil grew around Christ's tomb after He rose from the dead. It only came to Europe about 500 years ago.

The essential oils in basil make it one of the most calming and mood-enhancing of all the culinary herbs. Just keeping a pot on your kitchen windowsill will create an aura of peacefulness, even if you're cooking for 20. There are many different varieties: some with flat leaves, others that look as if they've been nibbled by rabbits, and some that have a very distinctive flavour. My favourite is purple basil – a wonderful addition to a simple spaghettini drizzled with extra-virgin olive oil and sprinkled with good Parmesan.

I've tried to grow basil, but sadly, without much success. It's quite sensitive to temperature changes and demands to be watered at the right time of day. Once you've got it going, however, you'll have delicious, fresh leaves for all of the summer as long as you keep picking out the young stems to encourage new growth.

Basil is too tender to grow outside during the winter, and many supermarket pots don't stay alive for more than a week; they're grown to have a short shelf-life. Unless you have a temperature-controlled greenhouse, you'll have to buy it fresh – but I think it's well worth it. The only other way to keep the fresh taste of basil in your kitchen throughout the year is to take the young leaves and add them to olive oil.

GARAM MASALA

Where would Indian cookery be without the spice mixture known as garam masala? Most of us in Europe assume that this is one basic spice ubiquitous to Indian cuisine. In fact, it has so many variations that it changes practically from village to village in India's northern provinces.

The most common form of this marvellous mix, which is used in Uttar Pradesh, combines cinnamon, bay leaves, cumin and coriander seeds, cloves, mace or nutmeg and black pepper. Other types add fenugreek, mustard seeds, cardamom and chillies. In some exquisite dishes, rose petals or a sprinkling of rose water are put in to provide extra fragrance – and they bring added peace to a wonderful spice mixture that already contains several anti-stress ingredients.

In the West, we normally associate garam masala with meat or poultry dishes, but I firmly believe that one of the great advantages of complex spices such as this is that they add good flavour to meals that some people might find slightly bland, such as vegetarian food or tofu.

One of the beauties of spice mixtures such as garam masala is that, although you can buy it ready-made, you can also make your own. After experimenting until you get the exact flavour you like, you can give your guests a dish that can justifiably be called yours and yours alone. If you make enough, it will keep in an airtight container for about three months. One thing to remember, however, is that no matter which combination you use, garam masala is best added just a few minutes before the dish is complete. If it's overcooked, you lose the wonderful aromatics of this subtle spice combination.

MACHO
FOODS

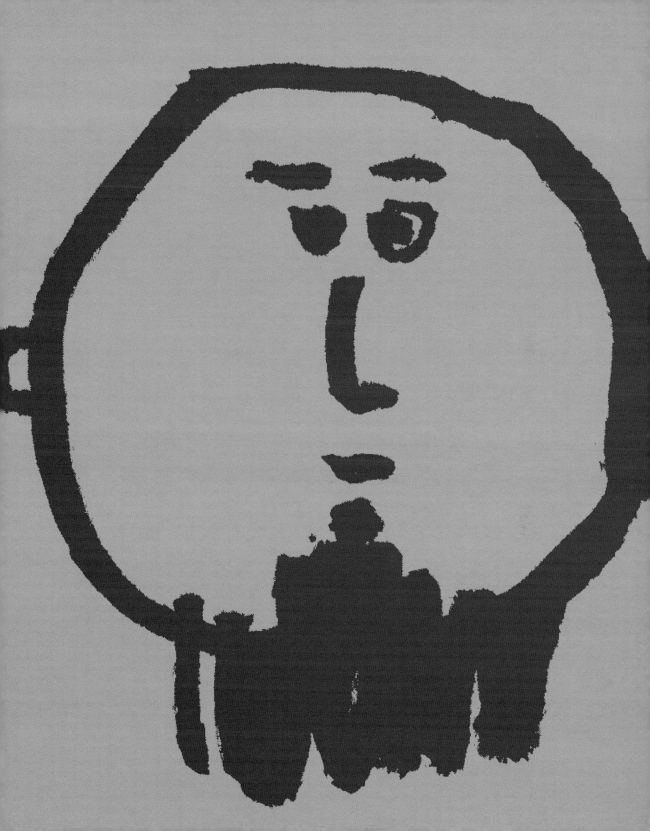

MACHO FOODS

Never before in modern history have there been so many challenges to man's sexuality. From a sociological point of view, many men are finding problems identifying their role in the male/female equation. Biologically, more couples than ever before are attending fertility clinics as a result of their persistent failure to conceive. Although there are many complex factors that contribute to this problem, one of the most obvious and most common is the ever-falling sperm count in today's men.

In fact, this vital prerequisite of conception has dropped by more than 50 per cent in the last 50 years. Despite the fact that there may be environmental factors (an ever-increasing level of female hormones in our drinking water; rising amounts of toxic material in food and drink), physical factors such as increasing obesity and the wearing of tight underpants and jeans, the major problem is simply poor nutrition.

Intensive farming methods have resulted in lower levels of zinc and selenium in our food. The first is vital for sperm formation, while the second is essential for sexual function. The minimum daily requirement of selenium is 70 micrograms (mcg) for a man, yet 20 years ago, the average intake had already fallen to 60mcg. Since then, it has halved. Today, the average British man gets no more than 30mcg of selenium from his daily food intake. Not only is this lack disastrous for sperm quality, it also seriously increases the risk of heart disease and prostate cancer.

The decline in selenium consumption is due primarily to EC regulations, which restrict the importation of flour from Canada and North America. There, the soil is rich in selenium, so crops grown in it contain higher levels. The majority of flour imports to the UK now come from Europe, where the soil contains far less of this vital mineral. In addition, bread consumption is declining, which explains the worrying drop in selenium levels in men.

Such statistics make healthy eating for men more essential than ever –
which is precisely why 'Macho Foods' are included in this book. Yet don't
stop here: apart from enjoying the following recipes, which include many
of the foods, herbs and spices renowned for their aphrodisiac and macho
benefits, every man in the UK would benefit from eating a few fresh,
unsalted Brazil nuts every day – just five provide the 70mcg of selenium
that are essential to a healthy diet.

Of course, many of the recipes contain ingredients that you wouldn't
instantly think of as being 'Macho Foods'. You Old Smoothie (page 112)
for example, makes use of peaches and mangoes, but these fruits play
a valuable role in manly health. Similarly, you may not think of garlic,
featured in Garlicious Soup (page 113) as an aid to your sex life, but
you'd be very wrong. It helps improve the circulation – and this, as you
must know, is a key factor in male sexual performance.

Oysters have a more universal reputation as an aphrodisiac, and the
muddy banks of the Thames are still littered with their shells. They aren't
that expensive, and are the best food source of zinc, which is why there
are two oyster recipes in this chapter: the Oyster & Salmon Booster
(page 115) and the Surprise Pie (page 118).

Tropical spices, such as ginger, chilli, cloves and turmeric; Tabasco sauce,
lean red meat and curry all have beneficial effects for male sexual health.
They improve blood flow, act as stimulants and, as a bonus, protect against
a range of illnesses, including heart disease and some cancers.

The dishes in this chapter are designed with men's health in mind, so
if you think your performance in the bedroom could do with a boost,
try them. You'll benefit from 'Macho Foods' – and so will your partner.

YOU OLD SMOOTHIE

At first glance, peaches and mangoes may not to be the most macho of fruits. Yet think about the Latin lovers and their passion for peaches, and the sensuality of South American tango dancers, for whom breakfast means mangoes. These exotic fruits are a cornucopia of nutrients essential for every man's good health.

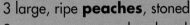

3 large, ripe **peaches**, stoned
2 **mangoes**, stoned and peeled
450ml or 16fl oz plain **bio-yoghurt**

1 Keeping aside one slice of peach and one of mango, put the rest of the fruit through a juicer.
2 Stir in the yoghurt.
3 Dice the rest of fruit finely, and serve on top of the juice.

CHEF'S NOTE: Many supermarkets these days keep soft fruit in a cold store, which ruins their flavour. Try to buy your fruit from a 'proper' greengrocer or local market.

GARLICIOUS SOUP

The term 'garlic-eaters' has derogatory overtones in today's society, but how wise such people are! Forget your phobia about the smell of garlic and boost your machismo with a big bowl of this soup. Garlic protects the heart, lowers cholesterol and improves circulation – and you know what that means. Add an extra boost from the ginger, and you could be in for a big surprise.

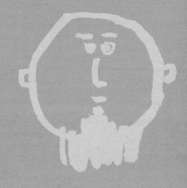

1 large head of **garlic**
4 tbsps **extra-virgin olive oil**
400g ᵒʳ 14oz **young courgettes**, trimmed but not peeled, cut in half lengthways and sliced
1 medium **potato**, peeled and finely diced
600ml ᵒʳ 20fl oz **organic vegetable stock**
1 medium **onion**, finely chopped
½ tsp ground **ginger**
2 tbsps toasted **pumpkin seeds**

1 Peel the garlic cloves, place in a roasting pan and roast in one tablespoon of the oil at 200°C ᵒʳ 400°F ᵒʳ gas mark 6 for 15 minutes.
2 Simmer the courgettes and potato in the stock for 15 minutes.
3 Soften the onion in one tablespoon of the oil. Add the ginger and continue cooking for two minutes.
4 Combine all the ingredients, including the remaining oil, in a food processor or mouli and liquidize.
5 Sprinkle with the pumpkin seeds and serve.

GREEN CHEESE PASTA

Sadly, many men regard avocados a bit like quiche: real men don't eat them. They couldn't be more wrong, however, as the high vitamin E content of these versatile fruits should make them a favourite of every would-be macho man. Lots of slow-release energy from the pasta, a circulatory boost from the Tabasco and ease of digestion make this a perfect lovers' meal.

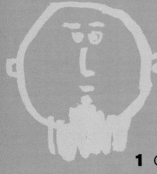

200g or 7oz **small pasta**, such as conchiglie
1 large or 2 small ripe **avocados**, stoned and peeled
175g or 6oz **mascarpone cheese**
4 drops **Tabasco sauce**
1 tbsp **coriander leaves**, finely chopped

1 Cook the pasta according to the instructions on the package.
2 Mash the avocado.
3 Stir in the cheese and Tabasco sauce and mix thoroughly. Thin with a little milk if necessary.
4 Pour the sauce onto the pasta. Season to taste, sprinkle with the coriander and serve immediately.

CHEF'S NOTE: This is a super-quick dish as there's no need to cook the sauce – the heat from the pasta is enough to warm it through. But you must serve it immediately in pre-warmed bowls; if it gets cold, the avocado will discolour and look like brown sludge.

OYSTER & SALMON BOOSTER

Quite frankly, I'm not a great oyster fan, but I love watching other people's obvious delight as they feast on these magnificent molluscs. Oysters are the richest natural source of the mineral zinc, essential for male sexual function. Just remember Casanova, who ate 70 a day, usually in the bath with his latest paramour. . .

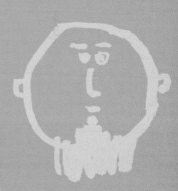

175ml ᵒʳ 6fl oz **dry white wine**
1 tbsp **light soy sauce**
1 tbsp **runny honey**
1 tbsp **capers**, soaked for 5 minutes in **milk**, then drained and lightly crushed
2 tsps **dried dill** or **fennel**
6 flat, round **native oysters**
280g ᵒʳ 10oz thin **salmon fillet**, skin removed and cut into bite-sized chunks
1 small bunch seedless of **black grapes**
1 bunch of **watercress**

1 In a saucepan, mix together the first five ingredients.
2 Warm through and allow to cool.
3 Prise open the oysters and add their liquid to the sauce.
4 Spoon the sauce over the salmon and oysters and chill for two hours.
5 Serve on a bed of watercress, garnished with grapes.

SPICY PORK CHOP

Ever since the days of the old City of London chop houses, this cut of meat has been a favourite with men. The heart-protection of garlic, the circulatory stimulants from the spices and curry paste and the healing enzymes in fresh pineapple add up to a perfectly masculine man's meal.

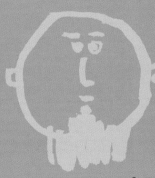

4 smallish **pork chops**
3 **spring onions**, finely chopped
1 **garlic** clove, finely chopped
3 tbsps **runny honey**
1 tsp **green curry paste**
½ tsp **herbes de Provence**
300ml or 10fl oz **organic vegetable stock**
2 slices **pineapple**, cut into chunks

1 In a frying pan, dry-fry the chops gently for three minutes each side.
2 Remove the chops from the pan and soften the spring onions and garlic in the juices.
3 Stir in the honey and curry paste, and cook for two minutes.
4 Mix the herbes de Provence with the stock. Add the mixture to the frying pan and warm through.
5 Place the chops in an oven-proof casserole dish. Pour the stock mixture over them and cook at 190°C or 375°F or gas mark 5 for 30 minutes.
6 Add the pineapple chunks 10 minutes before the end of the cooking time.

BEDOUIN LAMB

The strength, virility and ability to survive the harshest conditions are legendary among the Bedouin tribes – and nothing could be more manly than this dish. In addition to the protein harboured in the meat and beans, the cloves and turmeric – both traditional spices in Middle Eastern and North African cuisine – provide health-protective benefits against infections and some cancers.

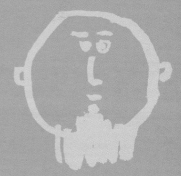

1 medium **onion**, finely chopped
2 **garlic** cloves, finely chopped
55g or 2oz **butter**
200g or 7oz **lamb fillet**, cut into chunks and rolled in **seasoned flour**
1 tsp ground **cloves**
1 tsp ground **turmeric**
425ml or 15fl oz **lamb** or **vegetable stock**
2 tbsps **sultanas**
115g or 4oz **broad beans**

1 In a large covered frying pan, soften the onion and garlic gently in the butter.

2 Add the lamb chunks and brown all over.

3 Sprinkle in the ground cloves and turmeric.

4 Pour in the stock and simmer for one hour.

5 Add the sultanas and broad beans and simmer for another half an hour.

6 Serve with boiled rice.

SURPRISE PIE

Surprise, surprise. . . more oysters for macho man. Of course, for other oyster-haters like me, this recipe is just as delicious without them – even if it does contain less zinc, an essential mineral for men. This dish's high protein content, along with plenty of iron, will keep any man red-blooded.

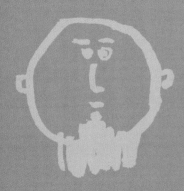

1 medium **onion**
3 tbsps **rape-seed oil**
350g or 12oz **braising steak**, excess fat removed and cut into small chunks
55g or 2oz **kidney**, trimmed and cut into chunks
2 tbsps **flour**
1 glass of **red wine**
85g or 3oz **mushrooms**, wiped and thinly sliced
6 **oysters**, opened and juice reserved (optional)
1 pack of ready-made **puff pastry**

1 In a large frying pan, soften the onion in the oil.
2 Add the steak and kidney and sear for two minutes.
3 Stir in the flour, a little at a time, and allow the juices to thicken.
4 Add the wine, cover and simmer for 40 to 50 minutes, or until the meat is just tender.
5 Mix in the mushrooms and oysters and simmer for five more minutes.
6 Pour into a pie dish, cover with the pastry and bake at 200°C or 400°F or gas mark 6 for 20 minutes.

TWO-FRUIT FLAN

Most men love desserts, yet many feel that they are 'off limits'. Here's the perfect compromise – a flan that looks good, tastes good and does you good. It provides huge amounts of betacarotene, which boosts natural resistance, is essential for good skin and is highly protective against some forms of cancer. There's also calcium, protein, B vitamins from the egg and a hint of brandy – just for fun.

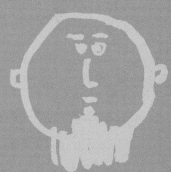

1 sheet of ready-made **shortcrust pastry**
125ml or 4fl oz **crème fraîche**
1 **egg**, beaten
1 tsp **brandy**
2 tbsps **brown caster sugar**
1 tbsp **plain flour**
200g or 7oz **apricots**, halved and stoned
200g or 7oz **figs**, halved lengthways

1 Use the pastry to line a 25cm or 10-inch tart dish. Bake blind at 180°C or 350°F or gas mark 4 for 10 minutes.
2 Blend the next five ingredients in a food processor or blender for two minutes, or whisk thoroughly by hand.
3 Arrange the fruit alternately on the pastry base. Pour over the liquid and bake for 45 minutes, until firm.

CHEF'S NOTE: This recipe allows you to use seasonally fresh fruit such as plums, peaches, cherries – or anything else that catches your eye. In winter, try it with soaked dried apricots.

MACHO HERB

DILL

This most delicate of frond-type herb has a long religious history. It is referred to in the New Testament book of Saint Matthew, where it was regarded as being so valuable that the Scribes and Pharisees donated it as an alternative to paying their taxes. In the colonial US, it was known as the 'Meeting House Seed', because children were given it to chew in order to stop them falling asleep and feeling hungry during over-long religious sermons. In medieval times, it was used to ward off the evils of witchcraft.

Dill also has a long medicinal history. It was used to cure coughs, headaches and whooping cough – and it's still the main ingredient in gripe water, used for decades to calm restless and fractious children. What most people don't know, however, is that this easily grown herb – a traditional accompaniment to simply roasted fish and part of the marinade for the Scandinavian raw fish dish gravadlax – was also added to wine to make both men and women more passionate; hence its use as a macho food. Dill stimulates the digestion, which is important if you're planning something adventurous shortly after a meal. It also encourages a healthy appetite.

Sown every few weeks in your garden or on pots on a balcony, dill will give you an abundant supply of fresh leaves for most of the summer. You can also leave some of the stems to flower and go to seed, drying the seeds for use throughout the winter. Use them in soups, with lamb stews and with any recipe that includes noodles or rice.

If you like giving homemade gifts as presents, try soaking some dill seeds in cider vinegar and pouring them into an attractive-looking jar. Your friends (especially the male ones) will be greatly impressed.

MACHO SPICE

GINGER

It may look like the most unappetizing of foods, but ginger is probably the most beneficial of all spices. These ugly roots (which are, in fact, rhizomes: thick, underground stems from which the plants reproduce) have been highly treasured in India and China for more than 3,000 years – with good reason, as we shall see below.

Ginger was one of the earliest spices to be brought to the Western world. The ground version was as common as salt and pepper as a condiment on late-medieval dining tables. Today, it is grown in many semi-tropical parts of the world, but Jamaican ginger – probably because West Indian cuisine uses it most – is widely regarded as the best type.

In Britain, it is still highly favoured as the ideal condiment to sprinkle onto ripe melon, while crystalllized ginger is put into rich fruitcakes. It is also used to make ginger wine, a wonderfully warming winter drink, and is the essential ingredient in that favourite childhood treat: gingerbread men.

Which brings us neatly to its macho associations. Like so many spices, ginger has been known throughout history as a great boost to the circulation. That is why it's particularly useful as an invigorating stimulant for men, particularly in the bedroom: it provides energy and get-up-and-go when it is really needed most.

Of course, ginger benefits women, too. It is a great cure for any sort of nausea, so take it if you're pregnant and suffering the awful pangs of early-morning sickness. Give it to the kids if they get carsick. And take a few cubes of crystallized ginger along if travelling makes you feel queasy.

SENSITIVE FOODS

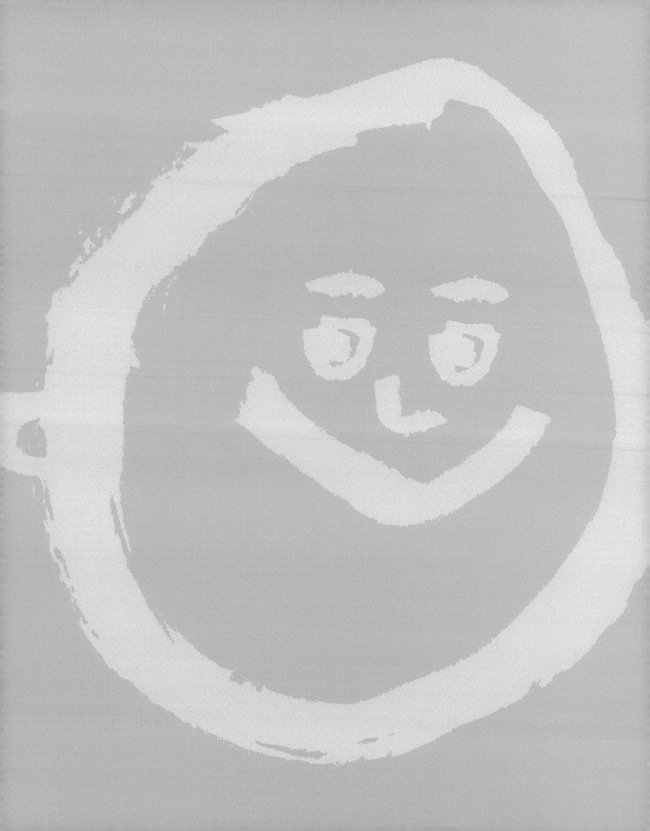

SENSITIVE FOODS

'Sensitive' might seem like a slightly wimpy and ineffectual way of describing someone in today's power-hungry, go-get-it world. Yet you only have to look at the number of counselling services available to realize that there are two sides to any person's character, and that both of them are necessary for a balanced life.

Of course, you have to have the confidence and strength to strive for the career you want, to succeed in a competitive hobby or simply to get up and face the world when everyone seems to be against you. Yet there are other times when, in order to be a good friend, an understanding colleague or a good manager at work, you need to be sensitive to other people's need. That means having a good insight into yourself, too.

It would be ridiculous to say that what people eat can magically transform them from ogres into agony aunts, yet there are foods that can keep you calm when the going gets tough. This is particularly important for women, who (unfairly, I would say) normally have to juggle several roles in their lives as well as deal with the regular rushes of hormones that can make any task seem so much more difficult.

The first essential rule to follow if you want to keep your emotional balance on an even keel is to make sure that you never go for long periods of time without food. If you find that the sensitive side of your nature seems to be constantly brow-beaten by uncontrollable irritation, anger and aggression, then this is a pretty good sign that your blood-sugar levels are suffering through erratic eating patterns. For many women, this state of affairs is made worse – again, uncontrollably – during their premenstrual days. For others, it forms a pattern that is quite unrelated to their hormonal cycles. If you recognize yourself in either of these descriptions, then now's the time to improve your eating habits and take advantage of the sensitive recipes on offer in this chapter.

The soothing enzymes in pineapple and the diuretic effects of celery and parsley in That's Cool! (page 126) are a great place to start. Next, try the strange-sounding but wonderful-tasting Smokie Soup (page 127). It's a magnificent mixture of kippers for brain-enhancing essential fatty acids and the mood-soothing benefits of oats – a truly sensitive soup.

Duck is probably not the first thing you'd think of for a meal that brings out the most sensitive side of your nature, but, surprisingly, it does, due to the fact that it is extremely rich in all of the B vitamins. In Turkish Duck Delight (page 132), you'll also find coriander and allspice – traditional spices of Middle Eastern and North African cuisine – both of which are famed for their ability to engender feelings of calm and sensitivity.

As many women have known for years, delicious desserts are the ultimate in romantic and sensitive foods. With this in mind, you won't find a simpler or more effective sweet than the Fired Apricots (page 133). The man in your life will usually get involved in any cooking project to do with fire – just try keeping him away from the barbecue – and the same is true of flambés. If you can tempt him into the kitchen, then he'll enjoy the romantic fun of cooking this dish for you. And you'll both benefit from the volatile oils provided by the star anise, which will, without doubt, leave you both feeling sensitive and romantic.

THAT'S COOL!

The cooling properties of cucumber are legendary, and it has been used for this reason in India's Ayurvedic medicine for thousands of years. Add the enzyme bromelain in pineapple, which helps digestion and speeds healing after any injury, plus the iron, vitamin C and antiviral benefits of strawberries, and this taste-tingling smoothie will help any woman keep her sensitivity and cool.

15cm or 6-inche piece of **cucumber**
4 **apples**
1 small **pineapple**, prickly leaves removed, sliced
1 medium bunch of **flat-leaf parsley**
125ml or 4fl oz plain **bio-yoghurt**
2 plump **strawberries**, cut into quarters

1 Run the first four ingredients through a juicer.
2 Stir in the yoghurt.
3 Pour into glasses, top with the strawberry quarters and serve.

SMOKIE SOUP

The locals on the Isle of Skye assure me that kippers and porridge aren't just for breakfast – and they're right. All the mood-soothing qualities of oats, omega-3 and -6 fatty acids from the kippers and the protective plant chemicals in garlic, leeks and onions make this surprisingly different soup a souper-booster for even the most non-sensitive of moods.

2 large **onions**, finely chopped
2 **leeks**, washed and finely chopped
1 **garlic** clove, finely chopped
1 fat **carrot**, grated
1 floury **potato**, peeled and grated
2 tbsps **extra-virgin olive oil**
55g or 2oz **unsalted butter**
4 skinned **kipper fillets**
85g or 3oz fine **porridge oats**
2 generous tbsps **double cream**

1 In a large saucepan, sweat the onions, leeks, garlic, carrot and potato gently in the oil and half of the butter for 15 minutes.
2 Pour in 850ml or 29fl oz water and simmer for a further 15 minutes.
3 Poach the kipper fillets in water and the rest of the butter for six minutes.
4 Flake the kippers and add to the soup. Stir in the porridge oats.
5 Leave to stand, covered, for at least 10 minutes. Serve with a dollop of cream in each bowl.

TENDERHEART'S TART

When your emotions have been trampled and you're feeling hyper-sensitive, a bit of self-indulgence doesn't hurt. In any case, the enormous health benefits of the onions and the emotionally healing aromatic oils in oregano or marjoram far outweigh the risks. A wedge of this, a glass of decent wine and a bowl of salad will heal even the most tender heart.

700g or 1lb 9oz mixed **red** and **white onions**,
cut into fine rings
60g or 2¼ oz **unsalted butter**
3 tbsps fresh **oregano** or **marjoram leaves**, chopped
1 sheet **shortcrust pastry**, baked blind for
10 minutes in a 23cm or 9-inch flan tin
3 organic **egg yolks**
6 tbsps **double cream**

1 In a saucepan, soften the onions very gently in the butter. Cover and continue simmering for 15 minutes.

2 Add the chopped oregano or marjoram leaves to the onions and simmer for 15 minutes more.

3 Pour the onion mixture into the prepared pastry case.

4 Mix together the egg yolks and cream, season with salt and black pepper and pour over the onion mixture.

5 Bake at 190°C or 375°F or gas mark 5 for 25 minutes.

PASTA PERSUASION

Serious discussions are always best held over a meal. For resolving conflicts, it's hard to beat this simple, delicately flavoured pasta. Basil's essential oils release mood-enhancing substances which act directly on the brain. Add the relaxing starches in penne and the zinc from shrimp, and you're bound to get your way with your dinner partner – wicked or otherwise.

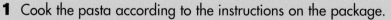

175g ᵒʳ 6oz **penne**
2 sprigs of **flat-leaf parsley**
20 sprigs of **basil**
3 tbsps **pine nuts**
2 **garlic** cloves
55g ᵒʳ 2oz **Parmesan cheese**, grated
150ml ᵒʳ 5fl oz **extra-virgin olive oil**
200g ᵒʳ 7oz **shrimp**, cooked and shelled

1 Cook the pasta according to the instructions on the package.
2 Place the herbs in the small container of a food processor and mix for 30 seconds, or chop them finely by hand.
3 Add the pine nuts to the herbs and mix again. Then add the garlic and cheese.
4 Add the oil gradually, mixing all the time.
5 Place the hot penne in a pre-warmed serving bowl. Add the shrimp, cover and leave for five minutes to warm through.
6 Mix in the pesto sauce and serve sprinkled with extra parsley.

FRESH SARDINE KEDGEREE

This unusual variation of traditional kedgeree is far removed from the stiff-upper-lip era of the Raj. Despite its robust flavours, you'll enjoy it in the most sensitive of situations. This is a particularly good dish for women, as it's rich in essential fatty acids for emotional balance, as well as providing vitamin D and calcium for strong bones.

2 **eggs**
675g or 1lb 8oz **baby spinach**
55g or 2oz **cooked rice**
115g or 4oz **Cheddar cheese**, grated
350g or 12oz **sardine fillets**, skinned

1 Beat the eggs and mix together with the spinach, rice and half the cheese.
2 Place half the mixture in an oven-proof dish.
3 Place the sardines on top.
4 Cover the fish with the rest of the rice mixture.
5 Scatter the remaining cheese on top and cook at 200°C or 400°F or gas mark 6 for 35 minutes.

CHEF'S NOTE: This recipe works equally well with any fresh, oily fish: fillets of mackerel, herring or pilchards, for example.

DEAR JOHN FISH

We've all had one or written one, so if a 'Dear John' letter is on your agenda, you'll need all the sensitivity you can muster. John Dory may be the ugliest of fish, but legend has it that the black spots on each side arose after the fish was touched by Saint Peter. True or false, this is certainly a dish blessed with the uplifting oils of oregano and the mentally essential minerals of the delicate white fish.

4 tbsps **extra-virgin olive oil**
2 tbsps **lemon juice**
2 tbsps **breadcrumbs**
½ tsp **dried oregano**
1.3kg or 3lb **John Dory**, filleted

1 Mix three tablespoons of the oil and lemon juice together. Stir in the breadcrumbs and oregano and season with salt and pepper.
2 Rub the mixture over the fish, cover and chill for one hour.
3 Drizzle the fish with the remaining oil and grill under a medium heat for 10 to 15 minutes each side.

CHEF'S NOTE: Don't be put off by the ugliness of this fish as it provides wonderful white fillets without any bones at all. You'll need one fish for two people and it's just as delicious pan-fried or baked.

TURKISH DUCK DELIGHT

I've always thought that the rich flavour of duck makes it an ideal food to share with a loved one. It's also a great source of emotionally supportive B vitamins. Cooked here with its covering of coriander, allspice and parsley, it provides a range of natural phytochemicals which help create feelings of emotional well-being.

½ a bunch each of **coriander** and
flat-leaf parsley, finely chopped
½ tsp ground **coriander**
1 tsp **allspice**
85ml or 3fl oz plain **bio-yoghurt**
2 **duck breasts**, on the bone, with skin
3 tbsps **rape-seed oil**

1 Mix together all the herbs, spices and yoghurt.

2 Smear the mixture all over the duck portions, pushing some of the mixture under the skin. Cover and chill for two hours.

3 Drizzle the duck breasts with oil and roast at 180°C or 350°F or gas mark 4 for 20 minutes.

4 Turn up the heat to 220°C or 425°F or gas mark 7 for 10 minutes in order to crisp the skin.

FIRED APRICOTS

Flambé dishes are wonderfully romantic, redolent of intimate, expensive restaurants and special nights to remember. The volatile oil estragol in star anise is mood-enhancing and calming, and the combination of eye appeal, wonderful smells and delicious taste makes this the perfect end to a romantic dinner à deux.

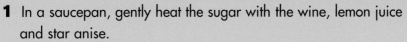

70g or 2½ oz **caster sugar**
125ml or 4fl oz **red wine**
3 tbsps **lemon juice**
2 **star anise**
25g or 1oz **butter**
6 ripe, medium **apricots**, left whole
3 tbsps **apricot brandy**

1 In a saucepan, gently heat the sugar with the wine, lemon juice and star anise.

2 Add the butter and stir over a gentle heat until it melts.

3 Add the apricots, cover and poach for 15 to 20 minutes, until the fruit is just tender.

4 In a separate saucepan, warm the apricot brandy over a low heat. Set it alight with a match and pour over the fruit.

5 Serve with double cream.

CHEF'S NOTE: It's easier to set fire to one large bowl of apricots, and serve it when the flames die down, but this dessert looks nicer if you bring in a tray of individual flaming bowls.

SENSITIVE HERB

OREGANO

This incredibly useful herb must have suffered several severe identity crises. Although its botanical name is Origanum, in different parts of the world it is known as marjoram, wild marjoram, winter sweet and winter mint, as well as many different varieties of oregano itself.

Whatever its name, I adore its slightly musty smell and flavour, and certainly wouldn't make a pizza without it. If I can't be bothered to make a proper stuffing, I just throw it into the cavity of a chicken with a few slices of lemon. I cut the young leaves and put them on pasta and into all manner of savoury pies. My wife says I'm obviously such a great fan that she's surprised I don't sprinkle it over my breakfast cereal. I love it, and I hope you will, too.

Oregano – and all its varieties – originated in the Mediterranean, and its name comes from the most beautiful Greek derivation. It actually means 'joy from the mountain', and it is still traditionally worn by both bride and groom to add an extra touch of romance when Greek couples get married.

More practically, oregano (and the rest of its family) is rich in thymol, which makes it an effective antiseptic. It also helps soothe colds, respiratory problems such as coughs and bronchitis, stomach upsets and seasickness. Most importantly, however, it helps to calm nerves, which makes it a wonderful herb for keeping you in touch with your own feelings and making you more sensitive and more open to other people's sensitivities.

SENSITIVE SPICE

ALLSPICE

At first glance, this spice may sound like a random mixture of all the exotic spices now available in this country, but in fact, allspice is a very specific, red-brown berry which originated in Jamaica. The berries grow on a flamboyant, evergreen tree which is abundant in the West Indies, yet it also grows well throughout Central and South America. The tree reaches almost nine metres (almost 30 feet) high and can live for an impressive 100 years. Its white summer flowers mature into green berries which are harvested, then dried and sold whole or, more often, ground.

Christopher Columbus first brought allspice to Europe, thinking that it was a variety of pepper. In Spain, it is still called *pimienta*, and you will also see it sold in English-speaking countries as Jamaican pepper.

Allspice is great to use in curries and rich fruitcake, and it adds extra flavour to exotic jams. It is also used commercially in pickles, ketchup and many other processed foods, such as sausages and pâtés. I always add a pinch to young rhubarb, and spend murky Sunday mornings making rhubarb, ginger and allspice jam.

Allspice contains a wide variety of essential oils – substances that give it its powerful, long-lasting aroma and that also contribute to its valuable therapeutic benefits. These naturally occurring oils, common to all the aromatic herbs and spices, have wide-ranging benefits, including mood-calming and emotionally enhancing properties. Some naturopaths believe allspice can also help with stomach disorders – but I'm not convinced.

EAT YO
HAP

URSELF
PY

GOOD MOOD A-Z

Have you come straight to the back of this book to look at these tables? You wouldn't be the first. After many years in practice and working in the media, I am certain that most people who buy health books, phone in to health programmes or send health queries to newspapers and magazines are primarily interested in specific conditions that affect themselves or their families. If you've come straight to these charts, you may not have noticed that this is a cookery book full of healthy, delicious recipes, every one of which has the added bonus of using one or more therapeutic ingredients.

These charts are not meant to be your sole method of diagnosis and treatment of whatever it is that ails you, but they do give you valuable guidelines about foods, drinks, herbs and spices that can all directly affect your mood. Many of the ailments described would not immediately spring to mind in relation to your mental state, but take a second look. After all, acne *is* stressful and depressing. Asthma *can* have negative emotional effects on young and old alike. Even recurrent cystitis interferes with sexuality and is a great source of anxiety, while PMS and fluid retention can be devastating emotionally. Few people realize that mouth ulcers, frequently recurrent and very uncomfortable, are more often than not related to stress, anxiety and low mood.

For these and other conditions, these charts will help. Here, you will find guidance and information about foods, herbs and spices that you should consume on a regular basis to help deal with the mood problems that may either be the underlying cause or a consequential symptom of any particular condition. It may sound simplistic that something as basic as changing your diet can directly affect your mood, but try it and find out for yourself. Go back to the beginning of the book, read the section most appropriate to yourself and make the suggested changes. With the help of these charts you really *can* 'eat yourself happy'.

Ailment	Food	Recipe
Acne	Cabbage and all its relatives are rich in sulphur. Fennel stimulates the liver and improves fat digestion. Garlic is antibacterial.	Poussin Parcels, page 38; Hushaby Herrings, page 52; Red Reveille Soup, page 65
Agitation	Basil and rosemary provide calming essential oils. Starchy foods such as pasta, rice, bread and potatoes offer brain-soothing tryptophan.	Squash, Tomatoes & Stew, page 19; Peacemeal, page 99; Laid-Back Lamb, page 103; Pasta Persuasion, page 129
Anaemia	Chicory is a good source of iron and the bitter flavour is an excellent appetite stimulant. Watercress contains iron and betacarotene and is highly cancer-fighting. Dates are a good source of iron for vegetarians. Red meat provides the most easily absorbed form of iron.	Bedtime Tea-Bread, page 57; Rare, Rich & Nutty, page 87; Oyster & Salmon Booster, page 115
Anxiety	Basil, chamomile, lavender and rosemary all contain soothing natural plant chemicals.	Granny Bly's Ice Cream, page 40; Chamomile Tea, page 146
Asthma	Onions, leeks and garlic all contain powerful natural chemicals which improve breathing and relieve congestion in this distressing condition. Avocado is a rich source of vitamin E, essential for healthy lung tissue. Watercress is a powerful natural protector of the lungs.	Sorrel-Leiki Soup, page 17; Green Cheese Pasta, page 114
Bloating	Celery and parsley are both cleansing and diuretic. Mint eases flatulence and improves digestion.	Pear-Power Punch, page 16; That's Cool!, page 126; Mint Tea, page 146
Blood-sugar problems	Carrots and potatoes, oats and beans all supply slow-release energy from the complex carbohydrates they contain. Dried fruits produce instant energy from their rich supply of fruit sugars, and a slower-release supply through the complex carbohydrates in apricot fibre.	Fishy Rice & Peas, page 22; Super Snoozer, page 48; Chicken Pick-Me-Up, page 71; Smokie Soup, page 127
Catarrh	Onions, leeks and garlic all contain powerful natural plant chemicals which improve breathing and relieve congestion. Watercress is a powerful natural protector of the lungs. Oregano's pungent aroma helps clear the sinuses and relieve catarrh.	Sorrel-Leiki Soup, page 17; Dear John Fish, page 131; Chicory & Watercress Salad, page 155

Ailment	Food	Recipe
Cholesterol	Garlic, chives and oregano help eliminate cholesterol and should be eaten regularly. Oats are rich in soluble fibre to keep cholesterol low. Apples and pears are also rich in cholesterol-lowering fibre. All dried beans are a good source of protein, fibre and energy.	Wakey-Shakey, page 64; Crustacean Couscous, page 69; Peacemeal, page 99; Garlicious Soup, page 113
Chronic fatigue	Basil, bay, lemon balm and sage help to improve mood and generate mental energy, the first step on the road to recovery. The next essential is the physical energy that comes from complex carbohydrates found in cereals, pulses and root vegetables. Protein from meat, poultry, fish, eggs and dairy products is the final ingredient.	Minty Potato Soup, page 33; Easy Cheese Frittata, page 34; Wise Old Fish, page 36; Smart Shepherd's Pie, page 39
Circulation problems	Basil, chives, coriander and sorrel all contain vitamins and phytochemicals which help stimulate circulation. Ginger and chilli have similar actions. Oily fish contain omega-3 fatty acids, and nuts and seeds provide vitamin E – both essential for a healthy heart and circulation.	Sorrel-Leiki Soup, page 17; Fishy Rice & Peas, page 22; Nutty Chicken, page 23; Passion Parlour, page 80; Garlicious Soup, page 113; Green Cheese Pasta, page 114
Colds	Garlic, chives and leeks have antibacterial and mucus-clearing benefits. Rosemary, sage and thyme are all powerful antibacterials and protectors of the mucous membranes. Cinnamon and cloves help relieve coughs. Pumpkin seeds and shellfish provide zinc to boost the immune system.	Savoury Polenta Cake, page 18; Fishy Rice & Peas, page 22; Peaceful Prune Pud, page 104; Oyster & Salmon Booster, page 115; Bedouin Lamb, page 117; Surprise Pie, page 118
Concentration problems	Liver's iron and B vitamins protect against anaemia. Garlic reduces cholesterol and improves blood flow to the brain. Sage enhances mental performance. Dried fruits provide quick and slow-release sugars to maintain a constant supply of essential sugar to brain tissue.	Spaghettini à la Vongole, page 35; Wise Old Fish, page 36; Hot Honeyed Prawns, page 37; Brazilian Brandy Pudding, page 41; Liver de la Nuit, page 55; Spicy Scrambled Eggs, page 66
Cystitis	Garlic has antibacterial and antifungal benefits – cystitis is often associated with thrush, caused by fungal infection. Celery and parsley are both natural and gentle diuretics. Drink plenty of fluids, especially cranberry juice.	Sleepy Sesame Chicken, page 53; Passion Parlour, page 80; That's Cool!, page 126; Pasta Persuasion, page 129
Depression	Basil helps the anxiety that often accompanies depression. Oats are rich in B vitamins. Bananas, liver and chocolate help increase levels of tryptophan, a gentle mood-enhancer.	Lullaby Lettuce Soup, page 49; Hushaby Herrings, page 52; Wakey-Shakey, page 64; Spicy Scrambled Eggs, page 66; Terrific Fruity Terrine, page 72; Smokie Soup, page 127

Ailment	Food	Recipe
Eczema	Pumpkins, red and yellow peppers, broccoli and sweet potatoes supply masses of betacarotene – essential for healthy skin. Wholegrain cereals offer B vitamins to help reduce stress. Oily fish provide anti-inflammatory essential fatty acids.	Squash, Tomatoes & Stew, page 19; Smoky Pasta, page 20; Tantalizing Tuna, page 21; Tofu Treat, page 98; Stressless Liver, page 101
Fever	Elderflower tea is particularly good for reducing temperatures during the daytime, while teas made from thyme, sage, oregano and marjoram all have antibacterial and antiviral properties that are useful in fighting fever. Garlic crushed with ginger and lemon juice is an excellent general remedy for fevers. Chamomile is one of the best anti-fever remedies for children – make a weak tea sweetened with honey and give two or three cups during the day and one at bedtime. An onion, baked in its skin for 40 minutes, then finely chopped and mixed in equal parts with honey, makes an effective remedy. Take a teaspoon or two every two hours.	Food isn't usually appealing when you have a fever. Once the temperature starts to fall, boost immunity and circulation with Spicy Scrambled Eggs, page 66
Fluid retention	Parsley is one of the most effective natural diuretics; add generously to cooking, as a garnish and in salads. It is also excellent as a tea; take two or three cups daily but not late at night as this causes sleep disruption. Celery is also gently diuretic and can be used in juices as well as raw or in recipes.	Sleepy Sesame Chicken, page 53; Passion Parlour, page 80; That's Cool!, page 126; Pasta Persuasion, page 129
Frigidity	Assuming there are no underlying psychological or serious medical problems, many foods may help: avocados, nuts and seeds for vitamin E; fish and shellfish for iodine; eggs for iron and B vitamins; tropical fruit for sexually enhancing enzymes; coriander, ginger and cayenne as traditionally sexually arousing herbs and spices.	Mangavo, page 81; Flirty Flan, page 82; Mussel Power, page 83; Turkish Duck Delight, page 132
Gastritis	Sage is astringent and cleansing to the gut; drink two cups of sage tea daily. Mint is an effective antacid and helps settle the stomach; use generously in cooking and drink as tea after meals. Cereals such as rice, couscous and oats are all soothing to the entire digestive tract. Live yoghurt contains beneficial pro-biotic bacteria, which improve digestion.	Wise Old Fish, page 36; Wakey-Shakey, page 64; Chickpea Trout, page 85; Dressed Breast, page 86

Ailment	Food	Recipe
Hair problems	Hair problems are always distressing, and can be helped by improving circulation to the scalp. Horseradish can be taken grated in a sandwich. Liver and red meat supply enormous amounts of iron and B vitamins which help with stress. Fish and shellfish are good sources of iodine for the thyroid (sometimes an underlying cause of the problem) and also provide many of the trace minerals required for healthy hair.	Three-Fish Carpaccio, page 84; Rare, Rich & Nutty, page 87; Laid-Back Lamb, page 103; Fresh Sardine Kedgeree, page 130
Halitosis	Fear of halitosis is a common cause of anxiety and withdrawal. Mouth problems are the most common cause, but indigestion and chest infections may also be a factor. Fresh, raw foods like apples, pears, celery and carrots all help to protect against gum disease, thanks to their fibrous nature. All citrus fruits supply vitamin C for gum protection. Herbs such as fennel, dill, mint and star anise are breath-fresheners. Plenty of live yoghurt maintains good digestive function.	Peaceful Punch, page 96; You Old Smoothie, page 112; That's Cool!, page 126; Fired Apricots, page 133
Headache	Headaches and good moods don't go together. Two common causes of headache are stress and low blood-sugar levels. Garam masala, rosemary, mint and basil are all traditional remedies for the relief of stress and its accompanying headaches. Liver provides iron and B vitamins – both stress-busters. Eating regularly will help maintain blood sugar on an even keel and prevent headaches caused by hypoglycaemia.	Peacemeal, page 99; Stressless Liver, page 101; Maori Chicken, page 102; Laid-Back Lamb, page 103; Skinny Dip, page 105
Heart disease	Garlic is a powerful weapon against heart disease, as it lowers blood pressure and cholesterol as well as reducing the stickiness of the blood. Eat at least one whole clove daily in food. Ginger, chilli and all curry spices contain phytochemicals which improve circulation. Wholegrain cereals and all dried beans also protect the heart by lowering cholesterol. Oily fish provide heart-protective fatty acids.	Passion Parlour, page 80; Three-Fish Carpaccio, page 84; Chard Chowder, page 97; Garlicious Soup, page 113
Heartburn	Mint is the most effective remedy of all. A glass of mint tea sweetened with a little honey after each meal and at bedtime will help relieve heartburn almost instantly. Rice is a traditional remedy for all digestive problems.	Fishy Rice & Peas, page 22; Minty Potato Soup, page 33; Peaceful Prune Pud, page 104

Ailment	Food	Recipe
Hypertension	Garlic is a powerful weapon against heart disease, as it lowers blood pressure and cholesterol as well as reducing the stickiness of the blood. Eat at least one whole clove daily in food. A cup of parsley tea two or three times daily is a good diuretic, which helps eliminate excessive fluid and thus lowers blood pressure.	Passion Parlour, page 80; Three-Fish Carpaccio, page 84; Chard Chowder, page 97; Garlicious Soup, page 113
Impotence	The minerals zinc and selenium are vital, and oysters, pumpkin seeds and Brazil nuts are some of the richest sources. Ginger, chilli, Tabasco sauce, cloves, turmeric and all curry spices improve peripheral circulation, which is vital for male sexual function.	You Old Smoothie, page 112; Oyster & Salmon Booster, page 115; Bedouin Lamb, page 117; Surprise Pie, page 118
Indigestion	Mint is the most effective remedy of all. A glass of mint tea sweetened with a little honey after each meal and at bedtime will help relieve heartburn almost instantly. Fennel and anise seeds are both excellent remedies for indigestion; use them to make tea and drink a cup after each meal. Rice is a traditional remedy for all digestive problems.	Fishy Rice & Peas, page 22; Minty Potato Soup, page 33; Peaceful Prune Pud, page 104
Infertility	Men should follow the advice under Impotence, but both men and women need an abundance of vitamin E. Eggs, oily fish and shellfish are all good sources of other nutrients important for female fertility, and the volatile oils in coriander also play an important role.	Passion Parlour, page 80; Flirty Flan, page 82; Mussel Power, page 83; Amorous Banana Split, page 88; Tofu Treat, page 98; Fresh Sardine Kedgeree, page 130
Influenza	Lavender helps relieve headaches associated with flu. Keeping up fluid intake is essential, and a mixture of hot mint and ginger tea with honey is an all-round soother. Turmeric and chilli both stimulate circulation and boost recovery. Live yoghurt, with its beneficial pro-biotic bacteria, is a mood-booster. Wholegrain cereals and oats provide B vitamins which help avoid the normal depression that follows flu.	Granny Bly's Ice Cream, page 40; Spicy Scrambled Eggs, page 66; Mangavo, page 81; Peacemeal, page 99
Insomnia	Lettuce provides natural plant chemicals that help induce sleep. Milk, starchy foods, turkey and oily fish offer soporific tryptophans. Nutmeg contains the mild hallucinogen, myristicin. Lime-blossom tea is a natural relaxant.	Lullaby Lettuce Soup, page 49; Cauli-Brocci Cheese, page 50; Sleepy Sesame Chicken, page 53; Tangy Turkey, page 54; Bedtime Tea-Bread, page 57

Ailment	Food	Recipe
Lethargy	Basil, bay, lemon balm and sage all help improve mood and generate mental energy, the first step on the road to recovery. The next essential is the physical energy that comes from complex carbohydrates, such as cereals, pulses and root vegetables. Protein from meat, poultry, fish, eggs and dairy products is the final ingredient.	Minty Potato Soup, page 33; Easy Cheese Frittata, page 34; Wise Old Fish, page 36; Smart Shepherd's Pie, page 39
Myalgic eucephalo- myelitis (ME)	Basil, bay, lemon balm and sage all help improve mood and generate mental energy, the first step on the road to recovery. The next essential is the physical energy that comes from complex carbohydrates, such as cereals, pulses and root vegetables. Protein from meat, poultry, fish, eggs and dairy products is the final ingredient.	Minty Potato Soup, page 33; Easy Cheese Frittata, page 34; Wise Old Fish, page 36; Smart Shepherd's Pie, page 39
Memory loss	Rosemary, the herb of remembrance, is an ancient remedy. Dried fruits and complex carbohydrates provide slow-release sugar. Oily fish and pumpkin seeds offer essential fatty acids which are vital for brain function.	Brazilian Brandy Pudding, page 41; Cauli-Brocci Cheese, page 50; Crustacean Couscous, page 69; A Fishy Caper, page 70; Laid-Back Lamb, page 103
Menstrual problems	Sorrel is rich in iron. Celery and parsley are both gentle diuretics and overcome fluid retention. Oily fish provides the anti-inflammatory effect of fatty acids. Dates offer extra iron. Bananas yield cramp-relieving potassium and vitamin B6, which help relieve PMS.	Sorrel-Leiki Soup, page 17; Savoury Polenta Cake, page 18; Sleepy Sesame Chicken, page 53; Bedtime Tea-Bread, page 57; Terrific Fruity Terrine, page 72
Mouth ulcers	These ulcers are nearly always the result of physical or emotional stress. Basil and rosemary provide calming essential oils. Starchy foods such as pasta, rice, bread, potatoes offer brain-soothing tryptophan.	Squash, Tomatoes & Stew, page 19; Peacemeal, page 99; Laid-Back Lamb, page 103; Pasta Persuasion, page 129
PMS	Sorrel is rich in iron. Celery and parsley are both gentle diuretics and overcome fluid retention. Oily fish provide the anti-inflammatory effect of fatty acids. Dates offer extra iron. Bananas yield cramp-relieving potassium and vitamin B6, which help relieve PMS.	Sorrel-Leiki Soup, page 17; Savoury Polenta Cake, page 18; Sleepy Sesame Chicken, page 53; Bedtime Tea-Bread, page 57; Terrific Fruity Terrine, page 72

Ailment	Food	Recipe
Restless legs	A common cause of insomnia and fatigue, often the result of iron-deficiency. Chicory is a good source of iron. Watercress contains iron, betacarotene and is highly cancer-fighting. Dates are a good source of iron for vegetarians. Red meat gives the most easily absorbed form of iron.	Bedtime Tea-Bread, page 57; Rare, Rich & Nutty, page 87; Oyster & Salmon Booster, page 115
Seasonal Affective Disorder (SAD)	Basil helps the anxiety that often accompanies depression. Hops are a powerful calmative and improve sleep quality; use them to make tea, or put dried hops in sachets inside your pillow case. Oats are rich in B vitamins. Bananas, liver and chocolate all help increase levels of tryptophan, a gentle mood-enhancer.	Lullaby Lettuce Soup, page 49; Hushaby Herrings, page 52; Wakey-Shakey, page 64; Spicy Scrambled Eggs, page 66; Terrific Fruity Terrine, page 72; these remedies only help to relieve the symptoms of SAD.; exposure to daylight or a light box together with the herbal remedy Hypericum (St John's Wort) should be used for the best possible results
Stress	Basil, chamomile, lavender and rosemary all contain soothing natural plant chemicals. Meat and poultry provide iron and a plentiful supply of B vitamins, which help combat the debilitating effects of stress.	Granny Bly's Ice Cream, page 40; Turkish Duck Delight, page 132; Chamomile tea, page 146; any soup made with organic vegetable stock cubes
Tired All The Time Syndrome (TATT)	Basil, bay, lemon balm and sage all help improve mood and generate mental energy, the first step on the road to recovery. The next essential is the physical energy that comes from complex carbohydrates such as cereals, pulses and root vegetables. Protein from meat, poultry, fish, eggs and dairy products is the final ingredient.	Minty Potato Soup, page 33; Easy Cheese Frittata, page 34; Wise Old Fish, page 36; Smart Shepherd's Pie, page 39
Thyroid problems	One of the most common undiagnosed problems in women. Underactive thyroid may be caused by a lack of iodine in the diet. All seafish and shellfish are good sources.	Hot, Honeyed Prawns, page 37; Crustacean Couscous, page 69; Oyster & Salmon Booster, page 115

GOOD MOOD DRINKS

Drinks are a great aid in the battle for good moods. Witness the great British cuppa, which seems to be the answer to every emotion. In times of happiness, we celebrate with tea. In times of stress, we make a stronger brew. In times of difficulty, we just add a few spoonfuls of sugar. Whether you're dealing with triumph or disaster, if you're British, out comes the teapot.

There are physiological reasons behind this tradition. Tea contains modest amounts of caffeine, loads of tannins and some important minerals, all of which have some effect on the mind and body. Yet if caffeine is something you'd rather avoid, or if you're simply not a tea-drinker, there are lots of natural alternatives which, in drink form, have an extremely rapid effect on your emotional state.

HERBAL TEAS

Both fresh and dried herbs can be turned into mood-altering teas. Most are made from leaves, although seeds can be used in some cases. If you're feeling stressed and anxious, try chamomile or lime-blossom tea. They're both available commercially in tea bags; simply add boiling water, cover, leave for five minutes, then add a little honey, if desired.

If insomnia's your problem, valerian or hops make ideal nightcaps, particularly if you add some honey as above. Use two teaspoons per cup of fresh herb, one teaspoon of dried. Both these herbs are very calming and help you to relax, thus making it easier to get off to sleep. Ideally, they should be drunk half an hour before bedtime and sipped slowly. If it's indigestion that's keeping you awake, then use a few sprigs of fresh mint, one teaspoon of dried mint or a commercial mint tea bag. The essential oils in mint are the best of all antacids, and will soon settle your stomach.

For instant vitality, especially during the winter months, ginger tea is a great energy-booster. The best way to make it is to peel and grate 1cm or 1/2 inch of fresh ginger, add boiling water, cover and let stand for ten minutes, then strain and sip slowly. If you find it a bit too strong for the palate, add one teaspoon of maple syrup or honey. Ginger has an instant stimulating effect on blood circulation, and you'll feel the difference within minutes of taking this delicious drink. As a bonus, ginger tea is also a great cure for travel sickness.

JUICES

For really interesting drinks, it's worth investing in a juicer. There is an excellent selection to choose from, such as Kenwood, Phillips or Moulinex, which start around £40.

For mood swings associated with the menstrual cycle, juice two or three apples, a stick of celery, a handful of parsley and three sage leaves, and stir into half a glass of soya milk. The sage and soya milk help regulate hormone levels, and the diuretic effect of parsley and celery gets rid of the uncomfortable swellings suffered by many women.

For a real pick-me-up, add three teaspoons of guarana extract to the juice of a mango, pawpaw, half a pineapple and two kiwi fruit. You'll gain a mountainous supply of vitamin C, along with masses of stimulating enzymes from the tropical fruits.

For romance, try this fresh-fruit cocktail. Juice 115g or 4oz each of blueberries and raspberries with 225g or 8oz strawberries and 225g or 8oz stoned cherries. The colour is glorious and the vitamins and minerals have just what you need to induce warm, amorous feelings. Top up with Champagne, if desired, for the best fizz you've ever drunk.

GOOD MOOD SUPPLEMENTS

I've used all the natural supplements listed below in my own practice for many years. They are effective and safe, and the best-quality products available. Broadly speaking, they fall into two categories: nutritional supplements that help maintain optimum levels of vitamins and minerals, and herbal remedies that have specific effects on mental and emotional functions such as memory, mood, concentration, vitality and energy levels. Remember: supplements are no substitute for a balanced diet.

VITALITY SUPPLEMENTS
Rio Trading Guarana: The traditional vitality-boosting herb of the Brazilian rainforest indians, which provides slow-release energy.
Ortis Ginseng: Rapidly absorbed liquid preparation of the Panax ginseng root.

BRAIN SUPPLEMENTS
Solgar Megadose Vitamin B Complex: B vitamins are vital for the normal function of the central nervous system.
Medic Herb Ginkyo: Standardized extract of Ginkgo biloba, valuable for the prevention of short-term memory loss, and may help slow the progression of Alzheimer's disease.

SNOOZE SUPPLEMENTS
Extracts of **valerian**, **hops** or **passiflora** help induce sleep.

WAKE-UP SUPPLEMENTS
Wassen Coenzyme Q10: Essential for converting food into energy. Good for chronic fatigue, Tired All The Time Syndrome (TATT) or ME.
Kelp: A rich source of iodine, which is essential for the normal functioning of the thyroid gland. Lack of iodine is a common cause of fatigue.

SEXY SUPPLEMENTS
Rio Trading Catuaba: South American aphrodisiac plant, used for centuries for the improvement of male sexual weakness.

Höfels Ginger capsules: Ginger is a powerful stimulant of capillary circulation, thus it is extremely useful in the treatment of male impotence. It's also valuable for women, as it improves blood flow to the genitals.

Seven Seas Oyster Concentrate with Zinc: Oysters contain zinc and other micronutrients that are essential for sexuality.

PEACE SUPPLEMENTS
Medic Herb Kava Kava: Standardized root extract that is mildly intoxicating and generates feelings of peace and happiness.

Kira St John's Wort: The great natural remedy for the relief of mild to moderate depression and the restoration of good mood. Avoid if taking immunosuppresents or blood-thinning drugs such as Warfarin.

Bio-Strath Elixir: Swiss herbal tonic with a wide range of proven benefits. Helps regulate mood, and is an ideal long-term mind/body tonic.

MACHO SUPPLEMENTS
Chilli: Powerful circulatory booster, improving blood flow, especially to the brain. Known to stimulate vitality and physical activity.

Wassen Serenoa C: Potent extract of the Saw Palmetto plant, a highly effective treatment for enlarged prostate glands. This problem is the most common cause of impotence and urinary difficulties.

SENSITIVE SUPPLEMENTS
Estroven: An excellent source of plant hormones extracted from soya beans. Helps regulate unpleasant symptoms of the menopause and may offer protection against osteoporosis.

Magnesium-OK: The ideal remedy for PMS, due to its content of magnesium, potassium and vitamin B6.

Evening Primrose Oil: When combined with Magnesium-OK, a daily dose makes the relief of PMS symptoms even more certain. There is also the added bonus of its benefits to the skin, particularly in the treatment of eczema.

GOOD MOOD AROMAS

The use of essential oils and their wonderful scents is at least 3,000 years old, and the value of aromatic oils and their perfumes cannot be over-estimated. From the Aztecs to the ancient Greeks, the Romans to the early Christian church, the mood-enhancing and medicinal properties of these oils have played a part in our civilization.

There are several ways of changing or enhancing moods by using aromatherapy. You can heat essential oils in a fragrancer, so that you breathe in their volatile vapours to achieve the desired effect, or you can dilute them with a vegetable carrier oil such as grapeseed, sunflower, corn or almond oil, and apply them to the skin. (When making up massage oils, use not more than a total of five drops of essential oil to each tablespoon or 5ml of carrier oil.) You can even add a few drops of essential oils to your bath water.

However, avoid direct application of all essential oils during pregnancy without professional advice, and never add thyme, basil, clove, cinnamon or peppermint oils to the bath, as they may cause irritation.

The following table matches essential oils to particular moods. The numbers refer to the total number of drops that should be added to one tablespoon of carrier oil.

VITALITY AROMAS
Massage: Lemon: **5**. Geranium: **3**. Frankincense: **2**
Fragrancer: Bergamot
Bath: Grapefruit

BRAIN AROMAS
Massage: Rosemary: **4**. Thyme: **4**. Basil: **1**
Fragrancer: Lemon grass
Bath: Fennel and juniper

SNOOZE AROMAS
Massage: Neroli: **4**. Geranium: **5**. Lavender: **2**
Fragrancer: Lavender
Bath: Mimosa

WAKE-UP AROMAS
Massage: Pine: **2**, plus juniper: **5**
Fragrancer: Eucalyptus and lime
Bath: Juniper

SEXY AROMAS
Massage: Rose otto: **5**. Jasmine: **3**. Sandalwood: **2**
Fragrancer: Sandalwood
Bath: Ylang-ylang

PEACE AROMAS
Massage: Ylang-ylang: **2**. Sandalwood: **3**. Bergamot: **3**
Fragrancer: Lavender
Bath: Orange

MACHO AROMAS
Massage: Cedar: **5**. Thyme: **2**. Cypress: **3**
Fragrancer: Sandalwood and cinnamon
Bath: Patchouli

SENSITIVE AROMAS
Massage: Jasmine: **4**. Lime blossom: **2**. Neroli: **2**. Carnation: **1**
Fragrancer: Jasmine and carnation

STRESS-BUSTER DIETS

People react differently to stress. Some lose their appetites; others turn to comfort eating and put on pounds, which causes even more stress. The recipes below contain stress-busting foods that are rich in complex carbohydrates, B vitamins for the nervous system and the antioxidant vitamins A, C and E for protection. At times of stress, your immune system may be severely depleted, which is why these protectors are so important. Take the time to shop and cook some of these dishes, and you'll be amazed at how quickly you start to feel better.

BREAKFAST
The most important meal of the day

Healthy English: Put one large mushroom, two extra-lean rashers of bacon, a tomato and a traditional low-fat sausage under the grill. While they're cooking, put a large plate on top of a saucepan of gently boiling water; when the plate is hot, break an egg into a cup then slide it carefully onto the plate, where it will cook without the need for any extra fat. Eat with a slice of unbuttered wholemeal toast.

Quick & Easy: Two slices of wholemeal toast, spread thinly with butter. Cover each piece with pre-sliced low-fat gouda cheese and a thinly sliced fresh tomato; pop it under the grill if desired. Partner this with a glass of fresh orange juice.

Porridge: Made with half milk, half water, porridge is the ultimate comfort breakfast and the best slow-release energy-provider there is. If you want to be really indulgent, stir in a dessertspoon of single cream just before eating.

Kippers in a Jug: Get a jug large enough to hold the kipper without the tail sticking out of the top. Fill with boiling water, and cover with foil. Leave for six minutes, remove and enjoy with a small knob of butter and wholemeal bread. Guaranteed to provide brain-nourishing essential fatty acids – without smelling up your kitchen!

SOUPS

Spicy Garlic Soup: Sweat 10 chopped garlic cloves and one chopped onion in three tbsps of extra-virgin olive oil until golden. Add one tsp crushed aniseed, and stir for one minute. Add 1 litre or 35fl oz water, bring to boil and simmer for 10 minutes. Add two slices of stale wholemeal bread and simmer for another 10 minutes, until the soup thickens.

Leek & Potato: Sweat one chopped garlic clove in 50g or 2oz butter. Add two chopped leeks, 375g or 13oz unpeeled, quartered small new potatoes, one sliced large onion and cook for 10 minutes. Add 900ml or 32fl oz organic vegetable stock and simmer for 20 minutes. Liquidize, then add 150ml or 5fl oz double cream, black pepper and two tbsps of finely chopped, fresh parsley.

MAIN COURSES

A fillet steak cooked with walnuts (*see* Rare Rich & Nutty, page 87) is an exceptional source of iron and vitamin B12. Perfect during times of stress, especially when combined with the minerals in the walnuts.

Fishy Rice & Peas (page 22): Cod and haddock contain protein, iodine and other minerals essential for peace and calm. The traditional West Indian rice and peas and classic combination of cereals and pulses encourage the brain's release of calming tryptophan.

Tangy Turkey (page 54): Turkey provides nerve-soothing B vitamins, marjoram encourages relaxation and a little rice wine ensures you enjoy a refreshing sleep after your meal.

DESSERTS

Brazilian Brandy Pudding (page 41): This unusual mixture of tapioca, milk, dried apricots and apricot brandy helps calm and relax.

Peaceful Prune Pud (page 104): This is rice pudding with a difference, perfect for stress control and for inducing sleep.

HAPPY WEIGHT-LOSS DIET

Crash diets don't work. They're not healthy, and it's impossible to get all the necessary nutrients on fewer than 1,000 calories a day. That said, there are times when people need to lose weight quickly: prior to an operation, for instance, or when excess weight puts severe strain on already damaged muscles, joints or tendons. Below is a five-day regime I've devised for my patients, with many years of success. Follow this healthy eating regime and you really can lose 10 pounds in 10 days.

DAY 1
Breakfast: Half a large melon.
Lunch: Vegetable soup or carrot and celery juice. A raw vegetable salad with brown rice and olive oil and lemon juice dressing.
Dinner: Mixed salad. Any cooked green vegetables with a well-rinsed can of your favourite beans (not baked) and one tsp of olive oil.

DAY 2
Breakfast: Freshly made apple and carrot juice, or fresh orange juice.
Lunch: Vegetable soup. A green salad. A baked sweet potato.
Dinner: A salad. Cooked green vegetables. Cooked cauliflower sprinkled with grated cheese and browned under the grill.

DAY 3
Breakfast: Half a grapefruit. An apple. Natural yoghurt with a little honey and chopped nuts.
Lunch: A baked potato with butter or one tbsp of sour cream and chopped fresh herbs. Coleslaw. A ripe pear.
Dinner: Vegetable & Cheese Casserole: wash and slice one green, red and yellow pepper, two courgettes, three tomatoes, one large onion, two garlic cloves. Rub a casserole dish with olive oil. Add the vegetables in layers, sprinkling each layer with a little olive oil, chopped parsley and basil.

Cover with foil. Bake at 180°C or 350°F or gas mark 4 for 45 minutes. Remove the foil. Sprinkle with two tbsps grated of Parmesan and bake until golden. Serve with steamed broccoli, and have an orange for dessert.

DAY 4

Breakfast: Porridge made with water and one tbsp of single cream. One slice of wholemeal bread or toast with a little butter.

Lunch: Winter Salad: mix shredded white cabbage, orange juice, four soaked dried apricots and two tbsps of chopped walnuts. Top with a dressing of two tbsps natural yoghurt, two tsps of runny honey and grated lemon rind. For dessert, have a stewed apple cooked with cinnamon and cloves.

Dinner: Watercress soup. Grilled Spiced Chicken: allow one skinned chicken breast per person. Chop one onion and a garlic clove and mix with natural yoghurt. Heat one tsp each of coriander and cumin seeds for two minutes. Crush and add to the yoghurt with half a tsp of chilli powder. Pour over the chicken and leave for one hour. Grill the chicken 10 minutes each side, basting with the marinade. Serve with steamed leeks and carrots.

DAY 5

Breakfast: Muesli with a sliced banana and a little single cream.

Lunch: A baked potato, with baked beans. Chicory & watercress salad.

Dinner: Carrot, Ginger & Orange Soup. Cod with Yoghurt Crust: place a large tub of natural yoghurt, one chopped onion, two garlic cloves, three tbsps coriander seeds, two tbsps of fresh mint, ground cumin, dried dill, paprika, plenty of nutmeg and two tbsps of chopped parsley into a blender. Place four cod fillets into a casserole dish. Pour over sauce and grill under a high heat, basting until a crust forms on the fish. Serve with a mixed salad.

NB: This diet can be repeated for another five days. Modest exercise will allow you to eat a bit more and enjoy a couple of glasses of wine a day.

ULTIMATE APHRODISIAC DIET

No magic foods or potions will make up for a life of continual stress, or compensate for a diet that doesn't provide enough protein, fats, carbohydrates, vitamins and minerals for healthy sexual function. On the other hand, many foods are reputed to have aphrodisiac properties, and adding these to your diet certainly can't hurt.

On the herbal front, a mixture of rosemary and hibiscus, for example, is a simple favourite. Tea made of this combination certainly has a romantic and sensuous perfume. The nasturtium, sometimes known as the 'flower of love', is not only delicious, it cuts a romantic dash as a decoration on your plate. An infusion of the fresh leaves — 15g ^{or} ½oz to 300ml ^{or} 10fl oz of boiling water — is said to have a mild stimulating effect.

Asparagus, figs, bananas, leeks, caviar, mushrooms and even hot spices are regarded as aphrodisiacs in some parts of the world, while other traditional strengthening foods for men include meat and eggs, aromatic herbs and sweetmeats made with honey. Chocolate's theobromine provides feelings of euphoria and happiness — just like being in love.

Scientifically speaking, the most important nutritional substances for normal sexual function are zinc, the B vitamins (B6 in particular), vitamins E, C and A and the trace elements selenium and chromium. One of the richest sources of zinc is the oyster, perhaps the most popular of all aphrodisiac foods (Casanova is said to have eaten at least 50 every day). Wheatgerm, oats and sesame and pumpkin seeds are also good sources of this vital substance, but they're all rich in vitamin E as well, so it's hardly surprising that they, too, are part of the sexy-menu story. If you want to turn your brief encounter into a romantic, loving and permanent relationship, then try the menu opposite.

THE ULTIMATE APHRODISIAC MENU

The Starter
A delicious dish full of eye appeal which makes a guaranteed romantic overture

Celery, avocado, grape and pink grapefruit salad, topped with a dressing of raspberry vinegar, pink peppercorns, extra-virgin olive oil and a sprinkle of sesame seeds, and decorated with sprigs of fresh coriander.

The Main Course
A light and nourishing taste sensation which oozes with sensuous promise

Grilled salmon steaks with a green sauce of gooseberries and fennel. To make the sauce: sweat the gooseberries in butter until tender and remove them from pan, add a drop of Pernod to de-glaze the pan, then mix in low-fat fromage frais to make a sauce. Finally add the gooseberries and finely chopped fresh fennel. Serve with baby new potatoes boiled in their skins, steamed broccoli florets with thin strips of carrot, and a tiny watercress salad topped with walnut oil and lemon juice dressing.

The Dessert
Simple and sexy, especially when fed indulgently to each other

A bowl of fresh strawberries, and whipped cream for dipping.

The Encouragement
It simply has to be bubbles

Half a bottle of pink Champagne.

The Savoury
Set the mood

Soft music, candles, and the inevitable. . .

INDEX

Entries in **bold** are recipe names

Acknowledgments

No book is exclusively a product of the author's efforts. Without my wife Sally's endless hours in the kitchen creating and refining recipes, the tireless efforts of my secretary Janet Betley, the numerous phonecalls from Hilary Lumsden, the gentle encouragement of Margaret Little and the ceaseless support of my agent Fiona Lindsay, this book would still be a twinkle in the eye.